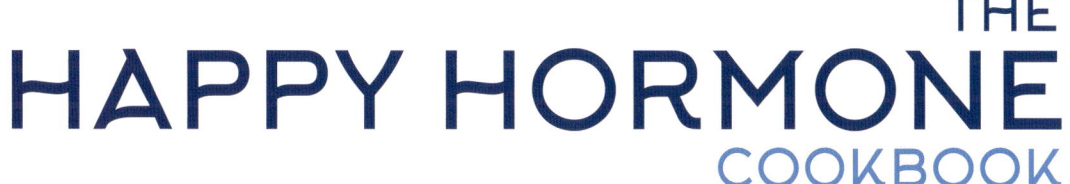

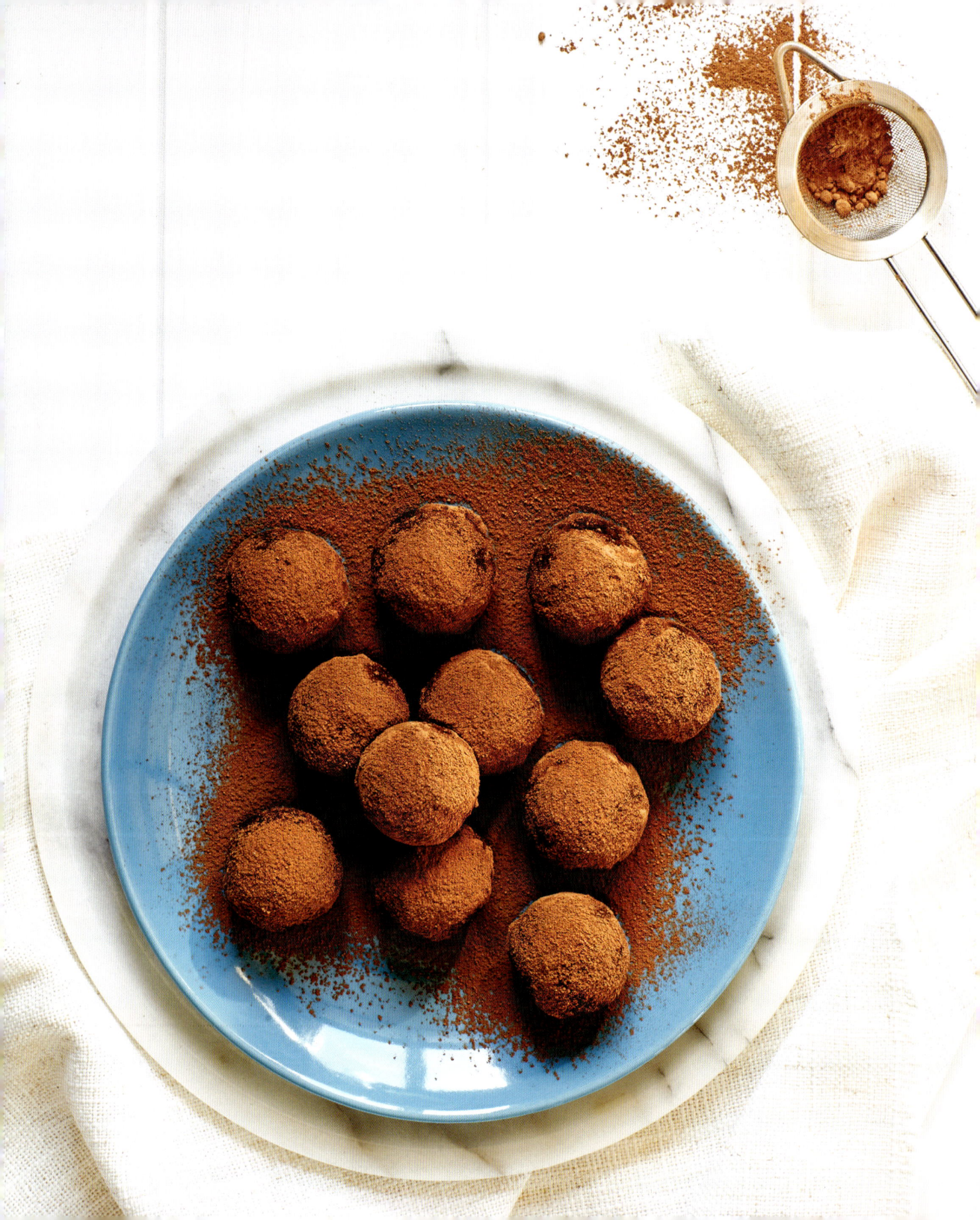

Food secrets for a balanced life

THE HAPPY HORMONE COOKBOOK

Emma Ellice-Flint with Jill Keyte

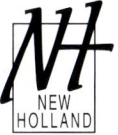

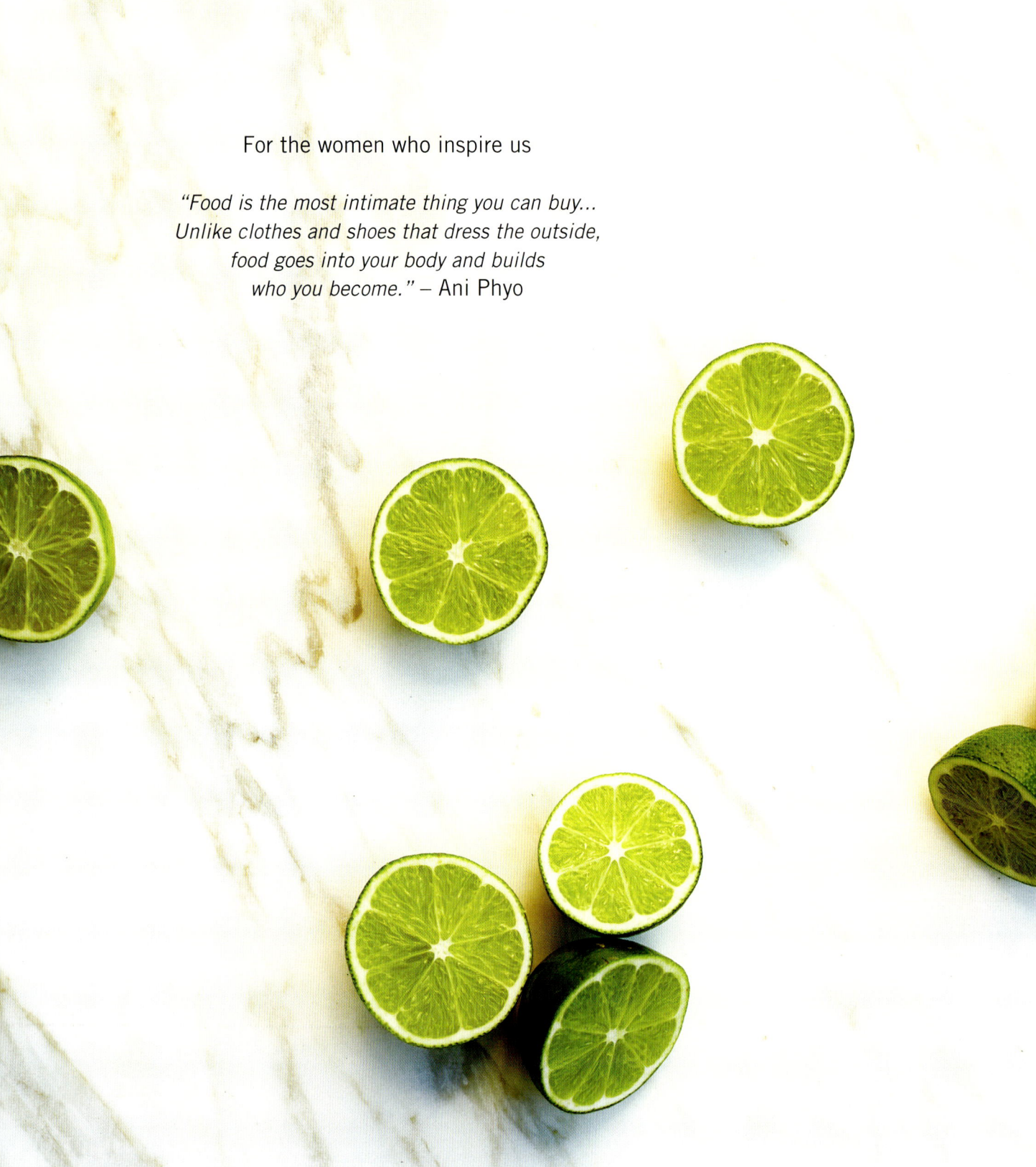

For the women who inspire us

*"Food is the most intimate thing you can buy...
Unlike clothes and shoes that dress the outside,
food goes into your body and builds
who you become."* – Ani Phyo

Contents

INTRODUCTION 7

Keeping your hormones happy 9

What is female hormone imbalance? 9
Alcohol 10
Anti-inflammatory foods 10
Balance 11
Bone health 12
Breakouts and maintaining the habit 13
Buying fresh and buying local 13
Digestion 14
Exercise and movement 14
Fiber 15
Flesh 15
Gardening 16
Good Fats 16
Grains 17
Gut health 18
Hormone disruptors 18
Liver Health 19
Mindfulness 20
Phytoestrogens and soy foods 22
Sleep 22
Stress 23
Sugar 23

How to make your own...
Bone Broth 26
Beef Broth 27
Nut Butter 28
Nut Milk 29
Flaxseed Meal 30
Sprouted Pulses 31
Home Cured Salmon 32
Labne 33
Pickled Turmeric Cauliflower 34
Pickled Ginger 35

Breakfast 37
Lunch 65
Dinner 101
Sweet things 139
Drinks 157
Snacks 171

Acknowledgements 187
Index 188
Profiles 190

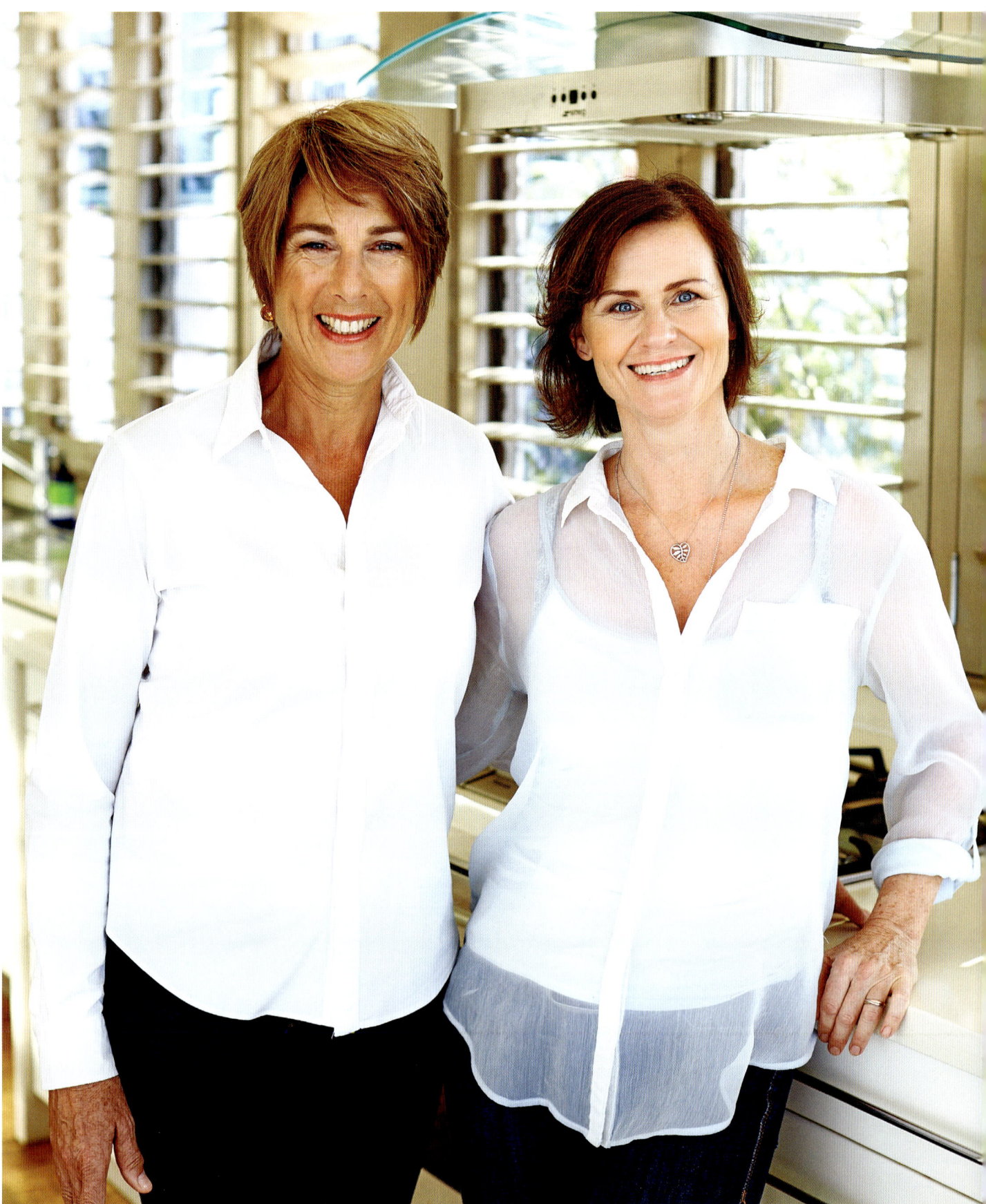

INTRODUCTION

We all have hormones – males and females. They change throughout our lives. Some females have painful and problematic menstrual cycles, others have difficult menopause, while many have little to no hormonal problems or side effects during their reproductive and post-reproductive years.

What we feed our bodies is important, no matter what our hormones are doing. All the recipes in this book are whole food recipes. They are predominantly plant based and full of phytonutrients and antioxidants. Most are naturally gluten-free.

Many of us are eating too much and the 'wrong' foods. We are not moving enough either. Combined with this, every day stress is a contributing factor to women finding themselves out of balance.

Perhaps you woke up one morning wondering where the person you used to be had gone. She used to have plenty of energy, had an upbeat outlook on life, a healthy weight and felt refreshed when she woke up. When this change occurs, it is often caused by hormone imbalance.

Emma works with people of all ages who are dealing with hormonal issues. She has written these nutritious recipes in response to her client's needs, conditions and requests. She has found that women who follow the ideas and eat from the recipes in this book can get more energy, better sleep, clearer skin, a healthy weight and elevated mood.

THINGS WE WANT YOU TO KNOW

- » Choose whole foods over processed foods. Whole food is food that has been refined as little as possible and is free from additives or other artificial substances.
- » Fresh is best.
- » Make it yourself.
- » Enjoy your time in the kitchen – on your own or with family and friends.
- » Love yourself and be kind to your body. You only have one, so look after it and it will look after you.
- » It's important to exercise daily. It keeps you vital, energetic and feeling good.
- » Take time out for yourself regularly.
- » Make it organic, whenever possible.
- » Grow your own. Gardening nurtures you and your harvest nourishes your body.
- » Small changes can have big benefits.

When choosing the recipes that we regularly cook at home, it is all too easy to stay in our comfort zone, to cook those things that are familiar or easy. We invite you to step out of this comfort zone.

If you start making some of the recipes in this book regularly, it will make a difference and will be worth doing. Not only will you love these foods, you may find your family and friends do too.

We have both been following the principles of this book for a number of years now and have learnt how to keep our bodies and hormones in balance. We do this through the foods we eat, our daily exercise, the management of stress and ensuring we regularly have time for ourselves. So we know the guidance we are offering here works.

Enjoy the benefits our recipes will give you. You may look and feel good as well as have more energy and vitality, feel sexy and proud. This book is for every woman.

Emma Ellice-Flint and Jill Keyte

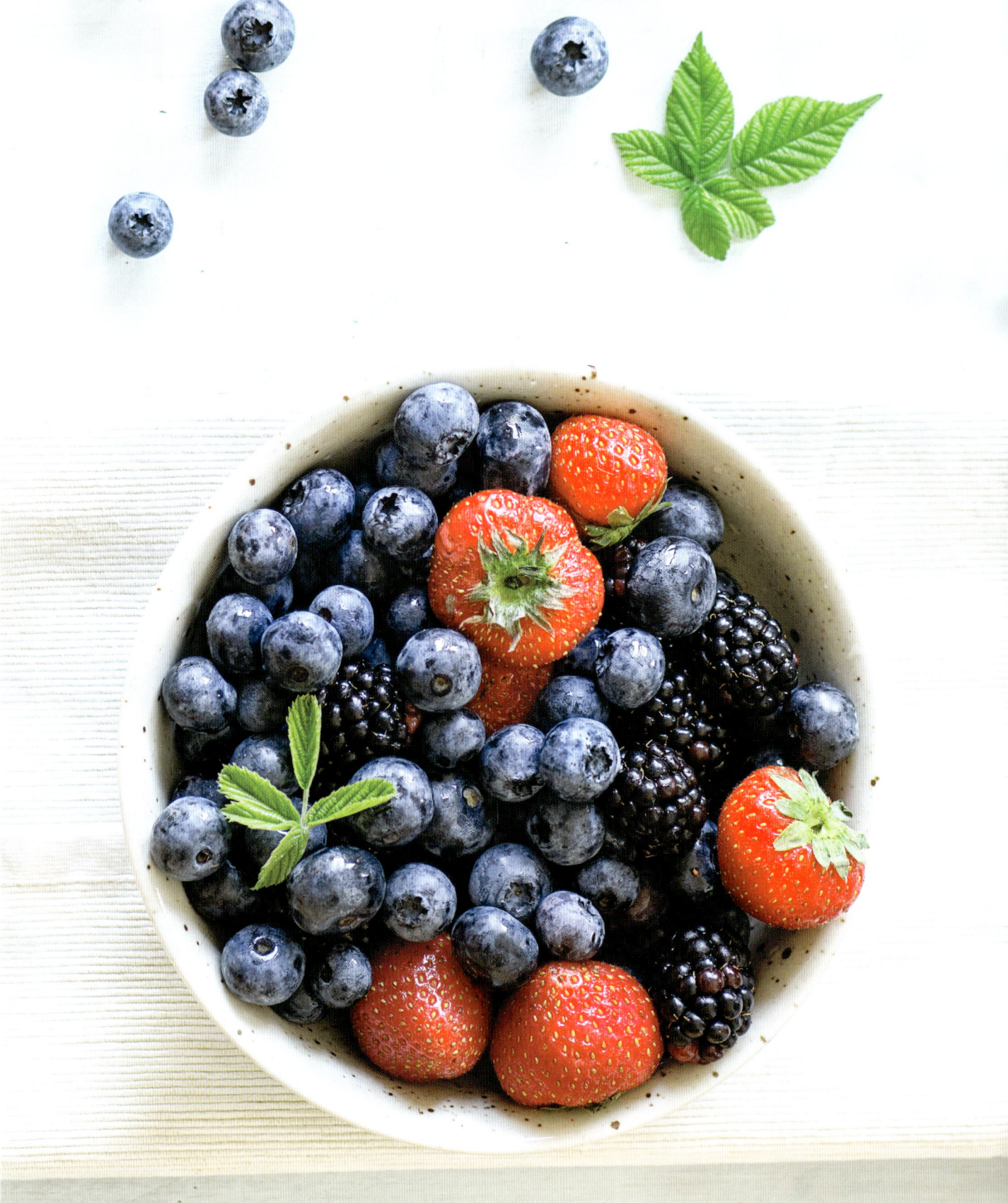

KEEPING YOUR HORMONES HAPPY

WHAT IS FEMALE HORMONE IMBALANCE?

A woman is unlikely to know when her hormones are in balance, but she will definitely know when she is out of balance. She may not associate the changes in her body or the symptoms she is experiencing with her hormones.

There are many symptoms of hormone imbalance including aching joints, change in bowel habits or disturbed sleep and Emma regularly finds in her clinic that these conditions are related in women of all ages. Some women can have a tendency to produce more oestrogen than is beneficial to their body. Others may have low progesterone giving them a higher proportion of oestrogen. Many of the foods in this book are designed to assist the body to eliminate this excess oestrogen and bring the hormones into balance naturally. This does not mean that a woman who is low in oestrogen, as occurs in menopause, has her precious oestrogen excreted. It simply means she can balance the hormones she has.

Relative excess oestrogen can produce some of the following symptoms at different times of the month:
- » Tendency towards pain, redness and swelling
- » Water retention and bloating
- » Weight gain
- » Irritability
- » Anxiety
- » Allergy and skin problems, including acne
- » Breast tenderness
- » Tendency towards depression
- » Abdominal cramping

Relative excess progesterone can produce some of the following symptoms at different times during the month:
- » Reduced libido
- » Fatigue
- » Tendency towards depression
- » Hard to get excited about things
- » Low blood sugar
- » Water retention

For women who are peri-menopausal or menopausal, symptoms are varied, and each woman will experience it in her own way. It is a natural progression of a woman's life, and some women experience relatively few symptoms, while others may have some or all of the following:
- » Menstrual bleeding changes. In peri-menopause there can be a shorter or longer cycle, heavier or reduced bleeding, spotting in between menstrual cycles. In menopause there is no menstruation.
- » Hot flashes
- » Reduced libido
- » Vaginal tenderness and dryness during intercourse
- » More frequent urination, irritation or infections in the urethra

- » Incontinence
- » Body aches
- » Sleep disturbance
- » Fatigue
- » Cognitive changes, mental 'fog'
- » Mood changes and reduced self-esteem
- » Increased facial hair
- » Hair loss

Do not self-diagnose. It is important to talk with a qualified physician about your symptoms and to have them properly diagnosed.

ALCOHOL

Alcohol can negatively impact your female hormone balance and the optimal function of your liver, as well as prevent nutrient absorption from your gastro-intestinal tract.

Alcohol slows down oestrogen metabolism, which means your body takes longer to rid itself of unwanted hormones. A higher alcohol intake is associated with high serum oestrogens, which can lead to increased PMS and menopausal symptoms.

Alcoholic drinks also contain sugar, detrimental to female hormone balance (see Sugar page 23).

If you are experiencing hormone imbalance, reduce your alcohol consumption to 4 standard drinks per week. If you're serious about getting your hormones in balance, we recommend not drinking alcohol for 4 weeks.

For healthy women, if you want to have an alcoholic drink we recommend one standard drink per day and a maximum of 7 drinks per week. Not 7 drinks in one day. That is binge drinking and is detrimental to your liver.

ANTI-INFLAMMATORY FOODS

Localized short-term inflammation is a natural reaction to injury or infection in the body. However, chronic inflammation can lead to female hormone imbalance and weight gain.

There are some star players when it comes to anti-inflammatory foods and hormone balance. These are:
- » Ginger
- » Turmeric
- » Omega 3 oils found in seafood, flaxseed (linseed), walnuts and chia seeds
- » Phytonutrient flavonoids found in vegetables, fruit, herbs and spices, legumes, cocoa and teas

Ginger is a potent anti-inflammatory. Several studies have shown that eating about ¼ teaspoon of dried ginger (equal to about 1 teaspoon of freshly grated ginger) per day, in the days running up to your period and during the first few days, relieves menstrual pain. Research has shown it can be as effective as taking anti-inflammatory drugs for menstrual pain relief.

Ginger also appears to help with migraine relief and reduced menstrual bleeding. Its potent anti-inflammatory and antioxidant benefits can help to relieve symptoms of peri-menopause. To get a great ginger fix, try the Fig and Ginger Slice (recipe page 149), Nourishing Broth with Ginger and Wild

Mushrooms (recipe page 74) or Ginger and Edamame Turmeric Fried Rice (recipe page 93). Also consider making your own Pickled Ginger to toss into salads (recipe page 35).

Turmeric is an all round anti-inflammatory and antioxidant. In her clinic, Emma has seen great results using turmeric as a food and as a supplement in its active ingredient form, Curcumin. Because of turmeric's anti-inflammatory properties, it can be beneficial in conditions such as endometriosis, a female inflammatory condition, and with peri-menopause and post-menopause. It helps with optimal hormone balance by supporting the liver's processes.

During menopause, if joints and muscles ache or become inflamed, turmeric helps with these symptoms. Some of our recipes with turmeric include Watercress and Mango Salad with Turmeric Prawns (recipe page 105) and Salmon and Turmeric Broth (recipe page 98).

Omega 3 oils are a really useful anti-inflammatory for female hormone balance. Some key areas, which can benefit from consuming Omega 3 oils over time, are:
» Mild depression
» Hot flashes
» Menstrual pain
» Endometriosis risk

The best source, but by no means the only source, is oily fish such as salmon, herring and mackerel. For vegetarians the best source is flaxseed (linseed), walnuts and chia seeds. Many recipes in this book contain Omega 3 oils. Some you might like to try are Home Cured Salmon (recipe page 32), Overnight Berry Oats (recipe page 53), as well as Salmon and Turmeric Broth (recipe page 98).

Flavonoids are a group of phytonutrients which trigger antioxidant benefits and anti-inflammatory effects. They often provide the vibrant color in vegetables and fruits and can support our nervous and cardiovascular systems, reduce insulin resistance and cholesterol. Many of the symptoms of menopause, PMS and other related unwanted female reproductive symptoms can potentially be reduced by consuming foods and drinks rich in polyphenol flavonoids. Plenty of the recipes in this book contain flavonoids.

BALANCE

Balance is often talked about in relation to work/life balance. We are not only interested in keeping your hormones balanced, but are keen for to you have a balanced life.

What are the important ingredients of a balanced life you may ask? Fulfilling our 'needs' – work, financial, family, education, community, as well as what's 'good' for us – social, health, exercise, leisure and spirituality.

We are interested in mind/body/spirit balance. Having too much focus on our 'needs' can lead to stress and an overproduction of adrenalin and cortisol, which can make us sick.

Whilst it's important to fulfill our fiscal needs, have work satisfaction and to care for our families, it is also important that we care for ourselves. Many women often put others before themselves, which can have a cost physically, mentally and emotionally.

By caring for ourselves, we mean:
» Finding a healthy body weight.
» Feeding our body nourishing food.

- Limiting 'quick and easy' takeaway meals.
- Doing regular exercise that raises your heart rate, stretches and strengthens your body and helps you maintain flexibility.
- Taking time out to connect with yourself, whether it be going for a mindful walk, listening to beautiful music, meditating, having a massage, being in nature.
- Connecting with friends and family.

All of these activities help relieve the daily pressures we experience. By ensuring self care has an important place in our lives, we can find and experience balance.

"Too hard", you say. We invite you to take on doing one loving thing for yourself each day.

BONE HEALTH

Our bones are at their strongest in our twenties. Whilst they continue to regenerate, they become thinner as we grow older. By looking after our bone health through our adult decades, we have a greater chance of slowing the thinning process. Women who are post-menopausal are more at risk of experiencing thinning bones and bone fractures through osteoporosis. You can look after your bone health through your diet and exercise.

When we think of keeping our bones healthy, we often think of calcium as the most important nutrient. Although it is very important, there are other nutrients, such as magnesium, manganese, zinc, boron, vitamin D, C, A and K2 as well as prebiotic foods, sunshine and exercise, which all benefit bone health.

A diet low in vegetables can have a negative affect on bone health. Research shows that a higher intake of vegetables, herbs and fruit may reduce bone turnover, particularly in post-menopausal women.

Foods that are high in inulin have a prebiotic effect, increasing calcium absorption and bone mineral density, especially in adolescents and in post-menopausal women. Inulin rich foods include onions, garlic, bananas, leeks, Jerusalem artichokes, whole wheat, barley and asparagus.

Prebiotic foods encourage good bacterial growth in your large intestine. Calcium relies on these bacteria to help it pass through the gut wall.

Interestingly calcium, along with magnesium, seems to help reduce premenstrual symptoms.

Food sources high in calcium include whitebait, tinned salmon (with bones), tinned sardines (with bones), dairy foods—especially hard cheeses, dried figs, tofu, legumes, sprouts, parsley, green leafy vegetables, seaweed, tahini, almonds, sesame seeds, wholegrain wheat and buckwheat, globe artichokes, broccoli, eggs, and fresh and dried herbs.

Food sources high in magnesium include whole grains – especially quinoa, brown rice, barley and millet – green leafy vegetables, fresh and dried herbs, nuts and seeds – especially almonds and pumpkin seeds, cocoa, eggs and legumes.

Many of the recipes in this book contain these foods and therefore these nutrients. We suggest you try the Wakame Seaweed Salad with Crunchy Tofu (recipe page 94) and Ranch Eggs with Spinach (recipe page 55).

Vitamin K2 helps activate osteocalcin for stronger bones. It is found in good amounts in the Japanese fermented soybean food called Natto. Natto is hard to find in regular stores. In Australia it can usually be found in the freezer section of specialist Asian or Oriental stores or in Japanese restaurants. It is a fermented food and is an acquired taste that is worth considering. Research has shown that Japanese women who regularly eat Natto have a lower incidence of bone fractures.

Vitamin K2 can be found in smaller amounts in quality hard cheeses with a rind, such as Parmesan, Manchego and Gouda. If you need it, you may find it easier to take Vitamin K2 as a supplement.

Vitamin D aids bone growth, remodeling and calcium metabolism. It is produced in your body through exposure to sunlight. Up to 20 minutes a day in the Australian sun in the early morning or late afternoon is ideal to top up your Vitamin D levels.

Be aware that caffeine, found in coffee, chocolate, some teas, cola and energy drinks, increases the excretion of calcium, as does alcohol consumption. Enjoy them, but in moderation.

Exposure to cadmium, through smoking and cigarette smoke, can increase your chances of getting osteoporosis by 20 per cent.

If you are concerned as to whether you are producing enough Vitamin D, a simple blood test by your medical practitioner, will measure it.

BREAK OUTS AND MAINTAINING THE HABIT

Eating healthily and being mindful doesn't have to be hard work. It's really about knowledge, choices and habit.

Knowledge
Knowledge requires a little education, that is, understanding the value of foods and what they provide for your body. We aim to give you some knowledge through this book.

Choice
Choice is about what you are choosing to eat and how often. If you eat out regularly, you may not be aware of whether what you choose is nourishing. We ask you to use this recipe book as a guide in making your food choices, be it at home or when you are eating out. You'll notice there are a number of foods, which appear regularly throughout the book. They are great to choose from a menu too.

No doubt you'll want to breakout from time to time and have a high carbohydrate, sugar and/or fat meal. All is not lost if you do. Our recommendation is just that you don't do it too often. Enjoy it and go back to making a nourishing choice for your next meal.

Habit
If we're honest with ourselves, we know when we are eating foods that are not nourishing us. Ideally you will start making nutritious food choices a habit. How do you develop the habit? Take on listening to your intuition or 'gut feel', rather than your craving or taste buds. Your intuition will know what your body needs and what makes it feel good. It's rarely wrong. Soon you'll find you're in the habit of making nutritious food and drink choices.

BUYING FRESH AND BUYING LOCAL

Where our food is sourced from is just as important as what we eat. These days you can buy most fresh foods all year round although it's often hard to know what is in season, and how many food miles (the distance over which a food item is transported during the journey from producer to consumer) most of our food has traveled.

We recommend choosing what's in season when you shop and buying food that has been sourced locally.

That's food that has traveled as few food miles as possible and, ideally, hasn't been kept in storage for long periods of time.

We recommend buying local because:
- It's usually fresh and has higher nutritional value.
- It's good for our local growers because they are more likely to get a fair price, which helps them to continue to grow locally.
- It's good for the environment because it helps reduce your carbon footprint as less fuel is required to transport your food.
- It helps to keep food dollars in your local community and contributes to the overall health of that community.
- It fosters agricultural diversity. Small local farmers grow the more flavor driven and often fragile varieties of fruit and vegetables which do not travel well over long distances.

If you have a Farmers' Market in your community we recommend you make this your first shopping stop. You will generally be buying directly from the producer. You can't get much fresher than that.

DIGESTION

In The Vital You workshops, Emma often talks about the benefits of preparing your food and how it aids your digestion. Your saliva increases whilst you plan and prepare a meal. So your digestion starts long before you sit down to eat.

The way you chew, including for how long you chew, can significantly impact your digestion and your health. We've got a few tips for getting the most out of your food.
- Sit down at a table to eat.
- Try not to have any distractions around such as television, electronic devices, newspapers, magazines or books.
- Enjoy sharing your meal with others.
- Put down your cutlery between each mouthful.
- Take smaller mouthfuls.
- Chew what you have in your mouth for 20–30 times before swallowing to ensure that you digest the food properly.
- Swallow and empty your mouth before you take another bite.

Eating this way is good for your health because chewing enables your saliva to begin the task of breaking down your food for digestion. This means your food gets digested more easily when it gets to your stomach and the nutrients and energy it provides are more effectively absorbed in the small intestine. This ensures your digestive organs are not overworked.

Last but not least, you enjoy and taste your food more.

EXERCISE AND MOVEMENT

Movement, in all its forms, is important and is good for your body. If your day involves a lot of sitting down, get up and move – stretch, walk or jiggle your body – every 50 minutes. Put your timer on, if you're someone who gets engrossed in what you are doing.

Find the movement and exercise program that works for you. Do what you like doing. What you have fun doing. Whether it's playing sport, going to the gym, walking, running, pilates, yoga, dancing, whatever makes you feel good, make sure you do it around five times a week. A combination of resistance, interval training, strength building, balance and flexibility work are ideal. You may also want to consider non-weight bearing exercise, such as swimming or cycling.

There's a plethora of activities to choose from. 60 minutes a day is recommended for teens and a minimum of 30 minutes a day for adults. If you need, get some professional advice about what is right for you.

When you exercise, you are forced to breathe more deeply. By breathing deeply, we mean using your diaphragm, rather than the top of your chest, as we tend to do when we are anxious or stressed. When exercising energetically, the pace and depth of your breath usually increases. In pilates and yoga especially, the rhythm and depth of your breath is integral to your movement. Research shows that regular exercise and learning how to breathe deeply have proven benefits for relieving menopausal symptoms.

The expression "move it or lose it" is not a joke. No matter your age, regular movement and exercise will aid your digestion, keep your body moving and feeling well and will help improve your hormone balance and mood.

FIBER

Fiber from the foods we eat is what binds to hormone metabolites in the digestive tract and pulls them out of the body in the faeces, thus being helpful in clearing excess unwanted hormones like oestrogen.

In fact, high fiber diets have been recommended to those needing to lower their estrogen levels, which are often higher in women with premenstrual symptoms. High fiber diets also benefit peri and post-menopausal women by improving gut function, reducing mood disturbances, inflammation and clearing metabolites caused by stress.

Fiber in our foods helps to regulate food movement through the gastro-intestinal tract, keeping us regular. This helps to keep our gut wall in good condition so it can absorb the nutrients from our food.

Soluble and insoluble fiber (see Porridge Three Ways page 42) in our diets 'feeds' our beneficial bacteria in our gastrointestinal tract.

These bacteria provide numerous benefits to us including:
- » Production of vitamins.
- » Facilitating the production of 'good mood' neurotransmitter hormones, such as serotonin.
- » Maintaining the delicate balance between helpful colonies and pathogenic bacteria.
- » Keeping our gut wall healthy, so we better absorb the goodness from our food and less of the toxins.

Most of the recipes in this cookbook are high in fiber.

FLESH

There is a lot of debate about the pros and cons of eating flesh. Our suggestion is select fresh meat – beef, lamb, pork, chicken, turkey or game – and seafood.

The most important thing is to know the provenance of your flesh. We suggest you follow these guidelines:

Red Meat – Grass fed, from areas with healthy soil, is best. Avoid beef, lamb and pork that is feedlot fattened. Ask from where the meat is sourced before purchasing. It is better to eat fresh meat rather than pre-packaged and processed meats. Processed meats can have preservatives, which do not benefit your body and can be carcinogenic.

Chicken and Turkey – Organic or free range, with no preservatives, hormones or antibiotics in their feed, is best for you.

Seafood – Check whether it is farmed and from where it is sourced. It's important to buy seafood from pollutant-free clean waters, especially shellfish. Large fish can carry heavy metals and other toxins, particularly mercury.

Some countries have strict regulations for water quality and feed content for farmed seafood. It's a good idea to check that your seafood supplier sources from seafood farms which follow these guidelines. This seafood, along with small wild-caught fish, calamari, squid and shellfish, is ideal to keep your hormones happy.

Note: Large fish to be avoided are fresh tuna, Orange Roughy (Deep Sea Perch), Catfish (Basa), shark (Flake) and Swordfish (Billfish/Marlin/Broadbill) because they are higher in mercury and can act as a hormone disruptor in your body.

GARDENING

There are so many benefits to gardening, whether it's in a small space or large. It can be quite meditative and a great stress reliever. It is also good exercise and connects you with nature. It gives you the opportunity to nurture, admire and harvest, if you plant a herb and/or vegetable garden.

It's so easy to grow your own herbs and vegetables. You can do so in pots, in a small plot in your back garden or through sharing a larger space in a community garden. The flavor of homegrown herbs, fruit and vegetables is often so much better than anything you can buy in the supermarket. Jill says "I used fresh mint out of my garden in the Mint and Bean Salad with Polenta Chicken (recipe page 133). It was delicious."

If you haven't tried gardening, we invite you to give it a go, even if it's in a small way. There is so much assistance available through TV gardening shows, books, magazines, gardening clubs and online. Your local nursery is one of the best places to help you get started as well as provide tips along the way.

If you have children assisting you, they will learn so much about from where their food comes. Jill volunteered in a School Kitchen Garden last year and found the enthusiasm of the children for planting and sowing was a delight. Through it they became conscious of sustainability and eating healthily. Planting and harvesting is always a surprise and is so good for your wellbeing.

GOOD FATS

There has long been a lot of misunderstanding about fat. There are 'good' fats and 'bad' fats. This misunderstanding has led to the fat being removed from many foods over the last 40 or so years. To give low-fat foods flavor, sugar has been added. This has caused other problems. (see Sugar, page 23)

The 'bad' fats are trans or hydrogenated fats, which are a type of unsaturated fat that is industrially produced from vegetable fats. This may sound healthy, but trans fats have often been associated with an increased risk of heart disease, which is the leading cause of death worldwide, and is growing in women.

These fats are highly inflammatory within the body. Trans fats have a long shelf life and are commonly found in processed foods, takeaway food and store-bought pies, cakes, margarine and biscuits. It is important to check the label when purchasing processed foods.

From a female hormone perspective, excess saturated fats can prevent the body from converting a strong form of oestrogen into weaker forms. We recommend you try to avoid large amounts of saturated fat, such as cream and fatty meats.

Extra virgin olive oil is a standout in the good fat category. It contains phytosterols, which naturally lower 'bad' (LDL) cholesterol and are anti-inflammatory. A 2009 Spanish study found a Mediterranean diet, especially rich in extra virgin olive oil, was associated with higher levels of blood antioxidants. Interestingly, this antioxidant capacity was related to a reduction in body weight!

Don't be afraid to use it in cooking. The International Olive Oil Council says, "When heated, olive oil is the most stable fat, which means it stands up well to high frying temperatures. Its high smoke point 210°C (410°F) is well above the ideal temperature for frying food. The digestibility of olive oil is not affected when it is heated."

Make sure your olive oil is extra virgin olive oil. Regular olive oil can be diluted with other vegetable oils and will not have the same health benefits. Cheap vegetable oils offer your body no benefit. You may think extra virgin olive oil is expensive. Its benefits far outweigh its cost. Store it in a cool dark place in a glass or ceramic container and be mindful of its 'use by date'.

Omega 3 oils are great performers as well when it comes to female hormone balance. They are anti-inflammatory, reducing symptoms of pre-menstrual syndrome (PMS) and menopause and help with balancing your moods. The best sources are wild herring, sardines, salmon and mackerel. If you can't source fresh fish, buy canned or pickled. Omega 3 oils are found in smaller quantities in squid (calamari), oysters and mussels. These are a sustainable source. See Flesh (page 15) for seafood sources and Hormone Disruptors (page 18) for potential seafood pollutants.

GRAINS

Grains are included in the whole food way of eating. The grains we have used in this book are not highly engineered or processed grains

How much and what type of grains you can eat often differs from person to person depending on your level of tolerance.

Grains are numerous. Those that contain gluten, a protein that is great for making bread elastic, are wheat, spelt, barley, rye, some types of oats, kamut, triticale and faro. Other grains, kernels and cereals that do not contain gluten are rice, corn, millet, amaranth, quinoa, buckwheat, teff and sorghum.

Grains have their benefits. One of the star players is oats – whole rolled or steel-cut (not quick or instant) because they contain insoluble and soluble fiber. The soluble fiber is called beta-glucan which protects the other food you have eaten from fast digestion. This means your food is digested more slowly and you get fewer sugar spikes. We have included several porridges (see Porridge Three Ways page 42) and other oat breakfasts (see Pink Oats page 47).

Another star is quinoa, one of the few plant foods that contain all essential amino acids. Quinoa is particularly high in anti-inflammatory phytonutrients and fiber. Along with amaranth and buckwheat, quinoa contains good levels of magnesium, a mineral that is important for many processes in our bodies, especially for women experiencing anxiety and tension with Premenstrual Syndrome (PMS) and menopause.

Other grains such as whole wheat and barley contain the prebiotic, inulin, which feeds your good gut bacteria.

In a typical western diet, a person may eat toast and/or cereal for breakfast, a sandwich or pastry for lunch and pasta or a burger in a bun for dinner. There is wheat in every meal, which is not a balanced way of eating. Eating a variety of grains over the day and often replacing them with pulses (legumes) or extra vegetables can give your digestive system a break from processing grains. We have included a wide range of recipes in this book that will enable you to do that.

Note: If you are eating grains and find you have abdominal bloating, constipation, diarrhoea, abdominal cramps, unexplained weight loss or feelings of tiredness, then it is important that you see a medical professional. They can run tests, which will determine if any serious medical condition is causing these problems. If the tests do not show any abnormalities, then you may have non-coeliac gluten sensitivity, in which case you may feel better avoiding gluten grains. If this describes a member of your family, make sure they have tests.

GUT HEALTH

It could be said that the foundation of hormone balance and wellbeing is a healthy gut. Probiotic bacteria take good care of this vulnerable part of your body.

They do this because they have genes that produce small, fatty acids such as butyrate. The villi (tiny finger like projections) in your gut wall like butyrate, which feeds the villi, causing them to grow larger and more robust. The larger they are, the better they are at absorbing macro and micro nutrients, such as vitamins, minerals and phytochemicals. When they are robust, the villi are less likely to let in unwanted substances and we gain more nutrients from our food.

Western guts have lower bacterial diversity, due to two things: a more relaxed use of antibiotics generally, which kill both the beneficial and the 'bad' bacteria in our gut. The second is the prevalence of a typical low fiber diet, which contains little prebiotic food. This does not give the food the beneficial bacteria it needs to thrive and multiply again.

Prebiotic foods, which help feed our beneficial bacteria, include leeks, asparagus, garlic, onions, artichokes, endive, Jerusalem artichokes, salsify and pulses.

Probiotic foods, containing bacteria that love to help improve our gut functioning and protect against harmful bacteria, are found in every culture in the world. These include yogurt, fermented vegetables such as sauerkraut and kimchi; miso, natto, fufu, unpasteurized vinegars, quality cheeses, ayran; kombucha, lassi and kefir drinks.

The beneficial bacteria and prebiotic foods, along with your liver's function, are important for the metabolism and reabsorption of oestrogens.

An unhealthy, unstable gut can lead to infection, causing mild inflammation, without you even knowing it. This can lead to hormonal imbalance in your endocrine glands, weight gain and mood disturbances. So look after your gut by eating the beneficial foods in this book.

HORMONE DISRUPTORS

There is a lot of research about environmental toxins and their potential endocrine (glands which secrete hormones) disrupting actions. Endocrine disrupting chemicals interfere with the synthesis, secretion, transport, activity or elimination of natural hormones. This interference can either block or mimic hormone action, causing a wide range of effects.

For instance, Belgian observational studies from the early 1990s showed that Belgium had the highest dioxin pollution in the world, the highest incidence of endometriosis and the most severe. However, there are no epidemiological studies to date, confirming the link of one class of chemicals. Although oestrogen-like compounds, such as the toxins listed below, are suspected.

A wide range of substances, both natural and man-made, are thought to cause endocrine disruption. These include heavy metals – mercury, lead, cadmium and arsenic; pharmaceuticals, dioxin and dioxin-like compounds, polychlorinated biphenyls, DDT and other pesticides, as well as components of plastics, such as bisphenol A (BPA) and phthalates. Sometimes called xenoestrogens, they are found in many everyday products such as plastic bottles, metal food cans, detergents, flame-retardants, food additives, toys and cosmetics.

Persistent organic pollutants (POPs) have been shown to possess endocrine disruption activities through interaction with oestrogen receptors and thyroid function. They are a variety of chemicals, which are either man-made or accidentally produced in industrial processes. Organochlorine compounds, such as DDT are part of this group of POPs, and were banned in the late 1970s because of their toxicity. Fat solubility, persistence in the environment and bioaccumulation potential in tissues through the food chain, make these compounds very toxic. Human exposure to POPs occurs primarily through the consumption of animal fats like fatty fish, meat and dairy products.

So, where possible, choose organic meat, dairy and eggs or where the soil, water and feed is checked for these endocrine disrupting chemicals. For example, some farmed seafood companies check both their water purity and the food they use to feed the fish.

When shopping for convenience, try to choose canned products that state the plastic coating inside is BPA free. Or better still, choose glass or ceramic containers and avoid plastic wrapped food wherever possible. It is important not to reheat your food in a plastic container or when covered with plastic film.

If using cosmetics, where possible, choose brands that state they are free from parabens, phthalates, nanoparticles and synthetic fragrances.

Your liver works hard every day to remove your body's natural metabolic by-products, so you want to minimize the environmental endocrine disrupting chemicals, which cause your liver to work harder. They can also cause you to have symptoms of fatigue and depression.

The aim is to lower your toxic burden. Don't think you have to aim for 100 per cent avoidance, because that is impossible. Reducing some of the toxins, like avoiding perfume, except for special occasions, will make a difference.

LIVER HEALTH

Our liver is a busy organ. Our bodies are constantly eliminating and detoxifying and the liver plays a major part in this.

The liver is also involved in our mental wellbeing. Our stressors can elevate our stress hormone, cortisol. It is the liver's role to process and remove it from the body. Often body fatigue, pain, mood disorders and immune dysfunction are a sign the liver is stressed from excessive external and internal stressors and is unable to do its job as well as it needs to.

For example, if a busy woman, who has elevated oestrogen is drinking caffeine to keep going, using alcohol to relax and wearing fragrance make-up, then it is highly likely she will have a busy liver. This means any excess oestrogen produced may not be processed and removed from her body as well as it needs to be. The excess oestrogen circulating in her body is likely to cause PMS, acne, hair dullness, weight gain and menopausal symptoms.

It is so important to take care of your liver with what you eat and drink, what you put on your body and by minimizing the environmental impact on it.

Glutathione is an antioxidant that is made in our bodies and is particularly beneficial to liver detoxification. The precursors that help make it are found in a variety of vegetables, fruits and flesh.

In particular; asparagus, spinach, garlic, avocado, potatoes, pumpkin (squash), zucchini (courgettes), melons, peaches, grapefruit and strawberries contain Glutathione.

Cabbage, broccoli, Brussels sprouts and cauliflower contain compounds that trigger production of Glutathione.

Flavonoids found in cinnamon, turmeric and cardamom increase Glutathione production.

The mineral, selenium, high amounts of which are found in brazil nuts, is also needed to make Glutathione in our bodies.

The sulfur-containing amino acid, cysteine, on which production of Glutathione depends, is found in garlic, onions and eggs.

Altogether these foods provide the means by which our bodies can make and use Glutathione.

Interestingly, a 2007 study found that practicing yoga assists with the production of Glutathione.

In other wisdom boxes we talk about ways to help the liver, the fiber-rich foods to eat more of, external toxins and the impact of stress. These all influence your liver health.

MINDFULNESS

Mindfulness is talked about a lot these days. What is it? How easy is it? Is it good for you?

Firstly, it is the practice of bringing your attention to the internal and external experiences occurring in the present moment. At the deeper end of the spectrum, it is meditation. If that is what you want to explore, it can give you a wonderful connection with your inner self.

If you find it difficult to stop for any length of time, then mindfulness could be the ideal practice for you. It can be easy, with practice, and it is good for you, if you are willing to push the pause button. Mindfulness harmonizes your nervous system.

By mindfulness, we mean taking a moment to check in with how you are breathing – fast, shallow, deep, slow, rushed; to be aware of your surroundings and other people, hearing, listening, seeing and observing.

There are so many demands on our senses and time these days. Sometimes we can't remember what we did, ate, saw, experienced, who we met or what we did and said in the last few minutes. We are being bombarded with noise, people, devices and lots more.

Mindfulness, in our words, is the art of stopping or pushing the pause button and being present to:
- » Our breathing—breathing deeply and slowly, taking in our surroundings, looking at the sky and taking in its beauty and magnitude.
- » Our inner voice and what our body is telling us that we need
- » What the important people in our lives are saying
- » The moment and what it has to offer

There is so much magic around us. We just need to stop to see, feel and hear it, especially when in nature.

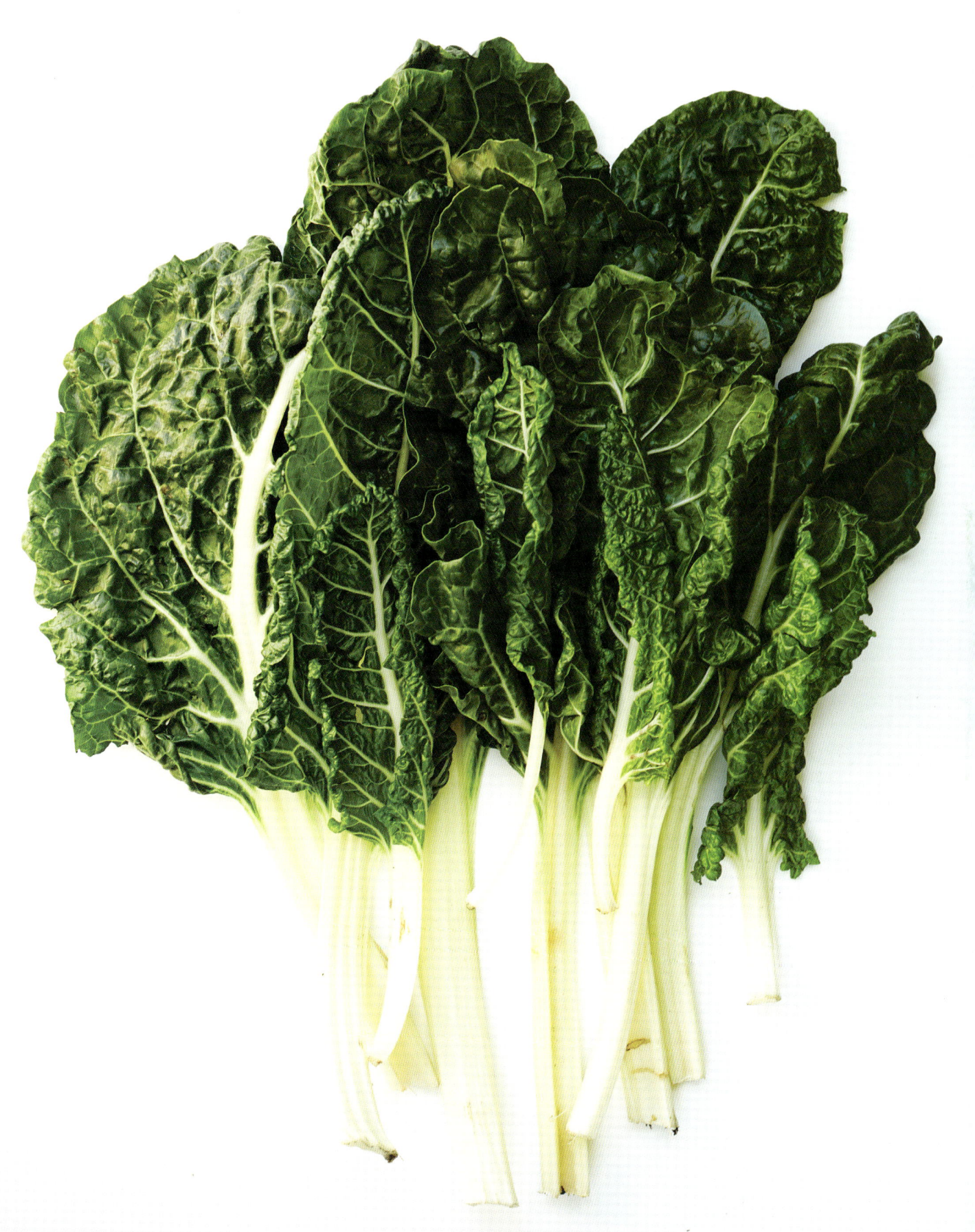

PHYTOESTROGENS AND SOY FOODS

Phytoestrogens are plant-based oestrogens that have the ability to occupy oestrogen receptors in our bodies. They can either enhance or modulate oestrogen activity naturally. This is of benefit whether you want to lower or increase oestrogen activity. However, they have a weaker physiological response than a woman's own hormones with dietary oestrogens being about 100–1000 times less potent.

Phytoestrogens are found in many foods, especially pulses eg. chickpeas (garbanzo beans), grains, olives, seaweeds and seeds, particularly flaxseeds (linseeds).

Phytoestrogens are also found in soybean foods, such as, roasted soybeans, tofu, tempeh, natto, edamame, miso and soymilks.

You'll find a lot of the recipes in this book have these phytoestrogen ingredients, because they are so good for you.

Phytoestrogen rich foods are good to have daily.

It is important to check what other ingredients soymilks and some tofu have. It is best to choose a brand that has natural ingredients, in addition to soy. If you can, take note of where the beans are grown and choose organic, as soybeans from some countries can be high in cadmium. Choose soy foods that list 'whole soy beans' as their soy ingredient as opposed to an isolate.

Start slowly, if you are introducing soy foods, and see how your body reacts. Some people can be intolerant or allergic to soy foods.

SLEEP

There are many reasons why someone wakes in the night, and finds it hard to return to sleep. This can be caused by high cortisol, low progesterone, high oestrogen, low serotonin, food sensitivity, gut issues, anxiety and poor sleep habits.

Over 80 per cent of serotonin, a neurotransmitter hormone involved in 'good' mood and sleep, is created in the gut. It is an intermediary in the production of melatonin, the 'sleep hormone'.

Foods that are of benefit to sleep are generally those that help reduce inflammation and boost gut function, which is the aim of every recipe in this book.

There is a 'bedtime dessert' that can help you sleep. Pumpkin seeds contain good levels of L-tryptophan. This aromatic amino acid is involved in raising levels of serotonin in the brain. Research indicates that eating about 35 g pumpkin seeds plus a high GI carbohydrate such as 30 g of dates, in the evening benefits sleep quality.

Pumpkin seeds are also a good source of magnesium, as are whole grains, green leafy vegetables, nuts and legumes. This calming mineral assists nervous system balance, and benefits sleep.

Make sure you get outside light exposure during some of the day, since this stimulates your production of melatonin, the 'sleep hormone'.

Being too warm, too cold, having a bright clock radio or electronic device nearby can affect the quality of your sleep. Small changes to your environment, the types of exercise you do, mind relaxation and room preparation can make a difference. All can lead to improved sleep quality. Jill uses a guided relaxation meditation to assist her to go back to sleep when she finds herself wide awake at 3.00am.

STRESS

Our lives seem to be getting busier. "I'm stressed", is regularly heard when you talk with colleagues, friends and family.

What is stress? It can be defined as a natural human response to real or perceived pressure when faced with challenging and sometimes dangerous situations. This pressure can be caused by what's happening around us. It is often caused by the demands we place on ourselves and let others place on us. We feel overloaded, tense, worried and anxious.

It is also when you feel the 'fight or flight' response regularly, even when we are not in danger. This can happen when you feel under pressure from work, deadlines, money, health and/or relationship issues. To compensate we produce the stress hormones, adrenalin and cortisol, in greater quantities. This can cause our bodies to go out of balance affecting our health.

If we keep pushing our minds and bodies when stressed, we can increase the production of our stress hormones to risky levels, with real physical impacts, such as:

- » Reduced libido
- » Poor skin
- » Suppressed immune system
- » Chronic fatigue
- » Unexplained infertility
- » Weight gain
- » Diabetes
- » Raised blood pressure
- » Increased risk of heart attack and stroke
- » Premature aging
- » Mental and emotional problems
- » Increased peri-menopausal symptoms

To power us 'out of danger', we often reach for a stimulant such as coffee, cigarettes or alcohol; high glycemic foods such as sugar and fast carbs, as well as give up some of our healthy habits.

There is 'good stress' and 'bad stress'. We like to call 'good stress' having motivating goals and challenges. 'Bad stress' can kick in when we lose our sense of balance. We can become addicted to busyness and stress. Is the potential downside worth it? When you feel stressed, we recommend you push the pause button, take stock, work out your priorities and ease the pressure.

Life is too short to spend it stressed. Whoever said at the end of their life, "I wish I'd spent more time working"?

You can have it all and we invite you to use this book to help you have it.

SUGAR

Sugar is a simple carbohydrate that comes in many different forms. The most common ones we consume are sucrose, lactose, and fructose.

How much sugar are you and your family having every day? Has it become an entrenched habit in your office or home?

According to the American Heart Association (AHA), the maximum amount of added sugars you should eat in a day is 25 grams (1 ounce) or 6 teaspoons for women. When you consider most soft drinks have at least 8 teaspoons of sugar, with sports drinks having significantly more, it is very easy to quickly pass the recommended daily limit.

Step back and check what your daily intake is. Look at the ingredients and/or nutrition facts on packaged foods for words such as sugar, glucose, maltose, dextrose, fructose and corn syrup. Where does it sit in the list of ingredients? If it is in the first three, it will have a high sugar content.

Most pre-packaged sweet foods are lacking in beneficial nutrients. When you eat them, you replace the opportunity of having more nutritious foods. Often you feel hungry again more quickly.

Our philosophy is, if you want to eat sugar, YOU should be in control of how much you have, rather than the companies and people who are making processed foods at a price, and for flavor, in preference to a concern for your overall health.

What happens to sugar in your body? When you eat sweet, low-fiber foods, they create a surge of blood sugar. Because your body doesn't like a lot of sugar in the blood all at once, it releases a flow of insulin from the pancreas. This is to tell the cells of the muscles, organs and renewing tissues to open up and take in the sugar. If they don't need it, the excess sugar goes to your liver packaged into triglycerides and cholesterol, then into your blood stream, making your blood 'stickier', and eventually to your belly. There, it is stored as fat.

Think of this repeated over and over again. Insulin having to 'knock on the doors' of your cells, increasingly having to knock louder, causing your pancreas to become exhausted. Mild inflammation is induced around your body. With regular over-consumption of sugar you may find yourself heading for metabolic syndrome – the main components of which are obesity, high blood pressure, high blood triglycerides, low levels of HDL cholesterol and insulin resistance – and a prediabetic state. Hormone issues are then caused by an overworked liver and chronic subclinical inflammation.

Let's also look at the emotional factors. There is a big relationship between the end of your menstrual cycle, that is around the time of your period, and a craving for sugar. Whilst you may crave sugar, eating foods high in sugar has been connected with a higher prevalence of Premenstrual Syndrome (PMS). These are hormonal events before a period that can cause side effects such as fluid retention, headaches, fatigue and irritability.

Over-consumption of sugar also alters the gut microflora and interferes with B vitamin absorption. B vitamins are used by the liver to carry out many of its processes, including mood regulation and energy production throughout our bodies. Are you peri-menopausal, with low mood and energy, feeling the need for sugar?

Instead of buying pre-prepared cereals, biscuits, cakes, soft drinks, muesli bars and other processed foods, make your own snacks, drinks and cereals! We have included a number of delicious options in this book.

At first it may seem hard to avoid sugar when you have been used to it. Go slowly on reducing it. Begin by taking out 'sugar drinks' you might have. Replace them with water. Sugar cravings can also be lessened by making sure there is adequate protein and 'good fats' in your main meals.

Batch-make savory snacks and have a healthy mid-morning and mid-afternoon snack instead of a sweet one. We suggest homemade hummus, which would be sugar-free, unlike some store-bought hummus (see recipe page 184), Rice Balls (see recipe page 174), Lentil Falafels (see recipe page 176).

This helps prevent a crash and craving. Also plan your meals, as it's best not to skip any.

WHERE TO SHOP

In some of the recipes in this book there are some unusual ingredients you may not have heard of before. We recommend the following sources.

- Firstly try your local shops. You will be surprised what is lurking around their 'health food', in the 'Asian' or 'international' sections. Alternatively try ordering online from a supplier that you trust.
- Umeboshi plums, miso paste, rice vinegar, seaweed, edamame, natto, buckwheat noodles and pickled ginger (unless you make your own, recipe page 35) – can all be found in Japanese or Asian or Oriental or health food stores.
- Amaranth, buckwheat, black rice, flax or linseeds and pulses are available from health food stores.
- Dried mushrooms can be bought from delis or providores, or Asian or Oriental stores.
- Cheeses such as Parmesan, Manchego and smoked hard cheese, as well as preserved lemons, Harissa and saffron, are often available from large delis or providores.
- Nuts and seeds are available in most large shops, but consider buying them in larger quantities direct from a company that specializes in them. Store them in the freezer. That way it saves you money and keeps them fresh.
- Extra virgin olive oil can be expensive, but is worth the money since it has far greater health benefits than regular oil. To help reduce the cost buy in larger amounts, perhaps direct from the grower if you can. Then share the oil amongst friends, splitting the cost. Make sure the extra virgin olive oil has a use by date, and that the oil's date is not close to expiry. The younger the oil, the more health benefits it contains.

HOW TO MAKE YOUR OWN

·Chicken Bone Broth (stock)· *Makes about 3–4 L (6–8 pints)*

Bone broth contains minerals, calcium and magnesium, which are very important, not only for bone health, but to aid the more than 300 chemical reactions in the body, including energy production and nervous system balance. Bone broth also contains gelatin. This is what gives the broth its thick liquid texture. Emma says, "there are lots of old wives tales about the powerful healing properties of chicken broth. I like these stories because, when I drink it, I feel it is nurturing, as well as nourishing me."

INGREDIENTS

- 3 organic chicken carcasses
- 4 large sticks of celery, washed and roughly chopped
- 2 large carrots, washed and roughly chopped
- 1 large red onion, peeled and roughly chopped
- ½ tablespoon apple cider vinegar
- ½ bunch parsley stalks (save the parsley tops to use in other dishes)
- 2 large sprigs fresh thyme
- 2 bay leaves (fresh or dried)

1. Place the carcass, celery, onion, carrot, vinegar, bay leaves and parsley stalks in a very large saucepan. Fill with cold water, close to the top, and well above the ingredients.
2. Place on the stove and bring to the boil without the lid on. It is very important to leave the lid off, otherwise your broth will go cloudy.
3. Turn down to a very low simmer so the water is just breaking with bubbles. Skim off any scum that has formed on the top. Don't worry if some of the cooking water comes off with this.
4. Allow to simmer for a minimum of 4 hours and up to 24 hours. The longer you cook it, the more minerals are released from the bones.
5. Once the cooking is finished, drain through a colander and allow to cool in a glass/stainless steel/ceramic container that will fit in the fridge. Leave the lid off. Once cooled, put in the fridge, with the lid on, and leave to go really cold. This allows any residual chicken fat to solidify on the surface, making it easy to remove. This is your base broth. If the flavor is a little light for your tastes, reduce it by boiling to intensify the flavor. Add some chopped herbs, if you wish.
6. To your broth you can add anything you want – finely chopped vegetables, shredded cooked chicken, cooked legumes, such as Borlotti beans. It is a great morning starter instead of a juice.

Note: Chicken carcasses are the bones that are left after the butcher has removed the flesh, legs and wings. There should be almost no flesh left on the bones. The chicken feet are also good to use. Ask your butcher to break them into smaller pieces, if you wish.

Beef Broth (stock)

Makes about 3–4 L (6–8 pints)

1. Buy organic beef bones from your butcher. Ask the butcher to cut the bones into smaller manageable pieces, about 5 cm (2 inch) long. This will enable you to get any marrow still clinging to the bones once they are cooked. The marrow is good for you and tastes delicious.
2. Before beginning the broth making, roast the beef bones for about 45 minutes in a hot oven, draining off any fat that has accumulated at the base of the pan. This fat is 'dripping' and, if you wish, can be used in cooking to replace oil or butter. You can also spread it on whole grain bread and eat it in the old fashioned way. If you wish, you can pull out and eat the marrow clinging to the inside of the bones.
3. To make your broth, follow the directions for making chicken broth.

Nut Butter *Makes 500 g (17 ½ oz)*

Nut or seed butter can be made with any combination of nuts or seeds. There are a few key things you need to know to make it super easy, rewarding and economical. The most common and delicious are almond, macadamia and cashew.

1. Set your oven to 150°C (300°F).
2. Warm 500 g (17½ oz) of raw nuts for about 5 minutes. This helps them to release their oils much faster and requires less grinding time. If you make less, it is hard work for you and your food processor.
3. If you want a roasted nut taste, then roast the nuts for a bit longer, about 10–15 minutes, depending on the size of the nuts. Make sure they don't over roast.
4. Place the warmed nuts in your food processor with a pinch of salt. Don't add any spices or herbs yet, as they can cause the mixture to coagulate and become sticky rather than a lovely creamy texture.
5. It can take 10–12 minutes, depending on the power of your food processor, to make the nut butter. If your machine becomes too hot or even smells of 'burning plastic', switch it off and wait for it to cool, before grinding again.
6. It is good to turn the machine off at intervals in order to scrape the sides of the bowl to make sure all the nuts are blending at once. Keep going with this process until you get the texture you want. If you want it crunchy, add extra nuts towards the end. It will be full of gorgeous good oils.
7. If you want to add other flavors, stir through when you have finished blending.
8. Store in a glass container in the fridge. It will keep for a couple of weeks.

Note: It is a great snack. See some options under Snacks on page 171 or Fig and Ginger Slice recipe page 149 and Orange and Cacao Balls recipe page 143.

Nut Milk
Makes about 1 L (33 fl oz)

This is very easy, and once you have done it, you'll wonder why you never bothered before. It is preferable to store bought nut milks, which often have added, unwanted ingredients to help them preserve and homogenize the milk.

You will need
- Food processor or blender
- Bowl or jug
- Large glass bottle or jar for storage
- Nut milk bag, muslin cloth or a very fine strainer. Nut milk bags are available from large kitchen shops or online.

INGREDIENTS
150 g (5 oz) raw almonds, hemp seeds or other nuts such as cashews
1 L (33 fl oz) filtered cold water
3 pitted fresh Medjool dates or 2 teaspoons pure maple syrup or honey or 3 teaspoons organic brown rice syrup
½ teaspoon vanilla extract or scraped vanilla seeds from half a pod

1. Soak the nuts or seeds in plenty of water in the fridge overnight. They will swell up. The next day, drain and rinse well.
2. Put all ingredients into your food processor/blender, and blend really well, about 2 minutes. Scrape down the sides. Then blend for another minute.
3. Sieve the blended mixture through the bag, cloth or strainer into a large jug or bowl. Squeeze or push as much juice as you can from the pulp. Then transfer the milk to the glass bottle/jar and store in the fridge or freezer. It will keep for about 4 days in the fridge.
4. As it naturally settles and separates, simply shake before each use.
5. You can use the leftover pulp in porridge, as crumble topping, tossed into salads or mixed up into dips.

Note: It is important you put the nuts into the fridge to soak, as you don't want them to begin their natural skin fermentation. Emma has made nut milk that has been left to soak on the kitchen bench overnight and, although it still makes great milk, it only keeps, even in the fridge, for a day or two before fermenting. And assuming you don't want this sort of fermentation, then she recommends soaking the nuts in the fridge.

⋅Flaxseed Meal⋅ *Makes about 60 g (2 oz)*

Flaxseeds (linseeds) need to be stored whole in the fridge and freshly ground for use. That way you can prevent their delicate oil from oxidizing and having a negative effect, instead of being a positive nourishing food for female hormone balance.

Flaxseeds are a rich source of dietary fiber, good oils, lignans and isoflavones. These provide soothing soluble dietary fiber, anti-inflammatory essential fatty acids, modulate oestrogen and help to reduce oestrogen reabsorption from the bowel.

---

1. To make your own ground flaxseed meal, simply put a small amount of the seeds into a clean coffee grinder or blender and grind into a fine meal. Alternatively use a pestle and mortar.

   Note: We recommend you use freshly ground flaxseed meal in these recipes. You can store any leftover meal for a couple of days in an airtight container in the fridge.

·Sprouted Pulses·   Makes 1 jar

There are many health benefits to making and eating sprouted pulses. They support your immune system and provide a diverse range of benefits, from improving your digestion to providing increased energy. In particular, pulses help support detoxification and elimination of any unwanted toxins and female hormones from the body.

By sprouting your own pulses you help to make the minerals, abundant in pulses, more easily absorbable.

Lentils and mung beans are the easiest to sprout. Although, mung beans do not taste as good as lentils. Of course, it is a personal choice. Puy and black lentils are best for sprouting. Quinoa and small seeds, such as alfalfa, also sprout well. The smaller the seed, the faster they sprout. Larger pulses, chickpeas/garbanzo beans can be crunchy and contain high levels of lectins, which can make your stomach bloat and feel uncomfortable.

Interestingly, research studies have shown that the absorption of beneficial nutrients in lentils is almost equal whether they are cooked or sprouted. I find them easy to sprout and love their delicious flavor and crunch in salads.

1. Soak one cup of (dried) lentils in water in a large glass jar overnight. They should fill about one-third of the jar. Cover with a tea towel or lid and leave on your kitchen bench.
2. Next morning, drain the lentils and wash them well a couple of times. Tip back into the washed glass jar so that they fill ⅓ of the container. Cover the top with a cloth, so that the lentils can 'breathe', and seal with a rubber band. You do not want insects getting in. Leave on your kitchen bench all day.
3. That evening, remove the cloth top, gently rinse the lentils and drain. Rinse the glass container; put the lentils back into it and cover and seal again. Leave on the kitchen bench overnight.
4. Repeat the rinsing and draining next morning and again in the evening. Depending on how warm your kitchen is, the lentils should begin to sprout by day three. Let them sprout until the root is longer than each lentil. Keep carefully rinsing and draining each morning and evening for 3–5 days.
5. Place the lid on the jar and put them in the fridge to keep fresh. They should last for a week.

Home Cured Salmon

Makes 1.5 kg (53 oz)

This is a great way to get your beneficial Omega 3 fish oils, which help reduce pain associated with menstruation and endometriosis and help minimize symptoms of menopause including mood.

You will need a large glass or ceramic container big enough to hold the salmon, (with the thin tail ends cut away). If you are nervous about curing a salmon for the first time, then start with one side of salmon or half of a side. Adjust the amount of curing ingredients appropriately.

Emma says, "I love the color of beetroot-cured salmon and really enjoy the flavor of dill-cured, so I have combined the two."

INGREDIENTS
- 1 fresh whole salmon, descaled, filleted and pin-boned, skin left on
- 60 g (2½ oz) unbleached sugar
- 50 g (2 oz) pure salt
- 1 tablespoon ground black/white pepper
- 1 bunch dill, washed and finely chopped
- 100 g (3½ oz) raw unpeeled beetroot, washed and coarsely grated

1. Put all the ingredients, except the salmon, into a bowl. Mix well.
2. Put one side of the salmon, skin side down, into the container and massage the beetroot cure all over it, in particular on the flesh side.
3. Massage more of the beetroot cure into the flesh of the second fillet. Place this on top of the first fillet, flesh side down.
4. If you have any curing ingredients left, pack it in and around the salmon so it is well covered, especially between the two flesh sides.
5. Put a lining of baking/parchment paper over the top of the fish. Place a small board (roughly the size of the salmon), flat plate or lid on top of the paper. Then place a heavy weight on top of this. Canned food is ideal.
6. If there's room put a lid on the container, otherwise wrap the container with plastic film.
7. Put the salmon into the fridge and leave it for 12 hours.
8. Take out of the fridge, drain off any liquid that has collected in the container and swap the fillets around, so the top fillet becomes the bottom one.
9. Repack the curing ingredients around the salmon flesh so it is well covered. Recover with the paper, board, weights and lid/wrap. Put it back in the fridge for another 12 hours.
10. Repeat once more. After 48 hours your salmon is ready to eat.
11. Scrape off the curing mix. It is fine to leave dill fronds that stick.
12. Using a large sharp kitchen knife, thinly slice the salmon almost horizontally, cutting the flesh away from the skin.
13. Store the salmon in the fridge for a couple of days or freeze in portions for later use.
14. Serve with avocado salad for lunch or for breakfast on rye toast with smashed avocado, lemon juice and 1 tablespoon of freshly ground flaxseed meal added to it.

·Labne· Makes 250 g (9 oz), about 12 balls

Labne is a yogurt cheese. It is high in protein and calcium with the yogurt giving it 'gut-loving' probiotics.

Equipment you will need:
- 30 cm x 30 cm (12 inch x 12 inch) clean muslin cloth
- wooden spoon
- bowl
- 500 ml (16 fl oz) glass jar

INGREDIENTS
500 g (17½ oz) natural unsweetened goat, organic cow or sheep yogurt (without thickeners)
Big pinch pure salt

250 ml (8 fl oz) extra virgin olive oil
1 garlic clove, peeled and crushed
1 sprig of rosemary, washed

1. Clean the jar thoroughly with hot soapy water, rinse and dry with a clean piece of kitchen paper.
2. Mix the salt into the yogurt.
3. Spoon the yogurt into the center of the muslin, gather and tie the corners, leaving a gap for the wooden spoon.
4. Put a wooden spoon through the gap and suspend the muslin ball over the bowl. Put this in the fridge and leave to drain. The liquid, which gathers in the bowl, is whey. You can use this in porridge, soups and smoothies.
5. After 48 hours, take the labne out of the fridge. Then, on a clean bench, open the muslin and roll it into balls, each weighing about 20 g (1 oz).
6. Carefully pile them into your clean jar. Add the garlic, rosemary sprig and the oil so that it just covers the balls.
7. Seal with the lid and store in the fridge for about a week to enable the flavors to develop before eating. You can store the labne for longer. If you wish to do this, make sure the jar is sterilized first before use.

Options:
- Emma likes to roll the labne balls in fresh finely chopped basil or parsley or cumin seeds.
- Use them with salads or spread on Sesame and Sunflower Crisp Breads (see recipe page 181).
- The leftover oil can be used in dressings or cooking.

Pickled Turmeric Cauliflower *Makes 500 g (17 ½ oz)*

In some traditional cultures, pickles are served along side every meal. Pickles help to stimulate your digestion and enhance the absorption of nutrients from your food. I have chosen to pickle cauliflower, a brassica vegetable, in this recipe, because brassicas have phytonutrients which enhance the function of your liver. This gives you a double benefit.

INGREDIENTS
500 g (17½ oz) fresh cauliflower
250 ml (8 fl oz) water
500 ml (16 fl oz) white wine vinegar
80 g (3 oz) unbleached sugar
1 heaped teaspoon turmeric powder
1 teaspoon black mustard seeds
½ teaspoon fenugreek seeds
A big pinch of salt

1. You will need a 2 L (4 pint) pickling jar.
2. Wash your jar and lid with hot soapy water, then rinse well. Put the jar into your oven to sterilize. Heat it to 120°C (250°F). Once it reaches its temperature, leave it in there for a further 10 minutes. Take it out carefully.
3. To sterilize your lid, submerge it in a pan of boiling water and leave for about 5 minutes. Take it out using tongs and wipe dry using clean paper towel.
4. Cut the cauliflower into small florets and pack them tightly into your jar, once it has cooled enough to touch.
5. Put the vinegar, water, sugar, salt and spices into a saucepan, bring to the boil and simmer until all the sugar has dissolved.
6. Pour the pickling liquid into your jar, filling it to just above the cauliflower florets, making sure every one is submerged. Aim to fill the jar to just below the rim, keeping a little space between the liquid and the lid.
7. Tap the jar to make sure no air bubbles are trapped between the cauliflower florets. Put the lid on tightly. Once the jar has cooled, put it into the fridge, and leave it for about 2 weeks to develop. It will keep in your fridge for up to 3 months.

·Pickled Ginger· Makes 75 g (3 ½ oz)

Ginger is incredibly good as an anti-inflammatory in the body, especially in the gut, where you want as little inflammation as possible. This helps your gut to absorb the nutrients from your food.

Make a small batch to begin with, so you gain confidence.

INGREDIENTS
1 large knob of fresh young ginger, about 75 g (3 oz)
1 tablespoon unbleached sugar
250 ml (9 oz) rice vinegar
1 teaspoon salt

1. You will need a 300 ml (10 fl oz) glass jar with a lid, washed thoroughly and dried with clean kitchen paper.
2. There is no need to peel the ginger. Wash it and trim off any ends that are dry.
3. Very finely slice the ginger with a mandolin, a food processor with a fine slicer attachment or a steady hand and sharp knife.
4. Put the vinegar, sugar and salt into a saucepan and bring to the boil, so that the sugar melts. Once the sugar has melted, add the ginger and turn off the heat. Mix it well. The ginger will go a subtle pink color. This is natural. In fact the younger your ginger, the more pink it will develop.
5. Pour into your clean jar and seal with a lid. It is ready to eat after 12 hours.
6. You can re-use the vinegar mixture for your next batch, once you have eaten all this one. Just boil up the vinegar mixture for a couple of minutes before using.

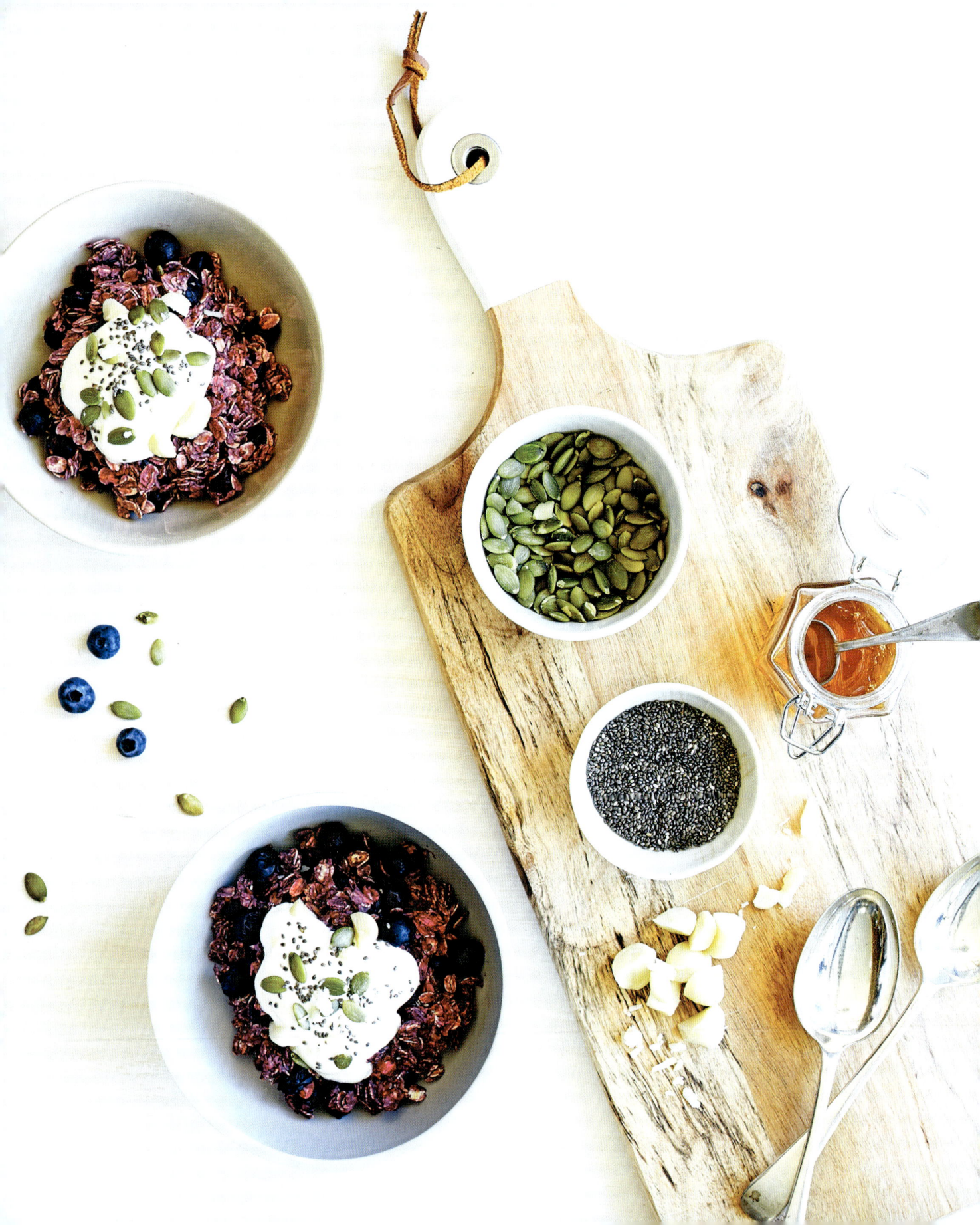

BREAKFAST

Black Rice Porridge
Serves 3–4

This chewy delicious 'porridge' makes a change from the oat-based versions. High in oestrogen clearing fiber, the black rice also contains the anthocyanin phytochemical (that gives it its black color). This provides both antioxidant and anti-inflammatory activity, helping our cell walls, especially our liver cells, to withstand stressors.

INGREDIENTS
- 200 g (7 oz) black rice, well washed
- 500 ml (16 fl oz) water, or whatever the packet instructions say to use
- 100 ml (3 fl oz) coconut milk
- 3 whole star anise
- ½ teaspoon ground cloves or 3 whole cloves
- 1 teaspoon cinnamon powder
- 1 teaspoon honey, pure maple syrup or 2 teaspoons brown rice syrup

Topping per person
- 2 tablespoons natural unsweetened organic yogurt
- ½ mango cheek, peeled and sliced
- 4 Brazil nuts, roughly chopped
- 12 almonds, roughly chopped
- 1 tablespoon flaxseed (linseed), freshly ground

1. Bring the water, spices, coconut milk, honey and black rice to the boil in a saucepan, then cook for one hour on low heat, or for the time specified on the rice packet.
2. When cooked, the rice will be soft and a bit sticky. You want to watch that the rice doesn't go dry during the cooking. Add more water, if necessary.
3. Remove the star anise and whole cloves. Spoon into breakfast bowls and stir through the ground flaxseed.
4. Top each serve with the yogurt, mango and nuts.
5. Place any leftover rice porridge in a sealed container and store in the fridge. It lasts a couple of days. Reheat as needed or freeze in individual sized portions.

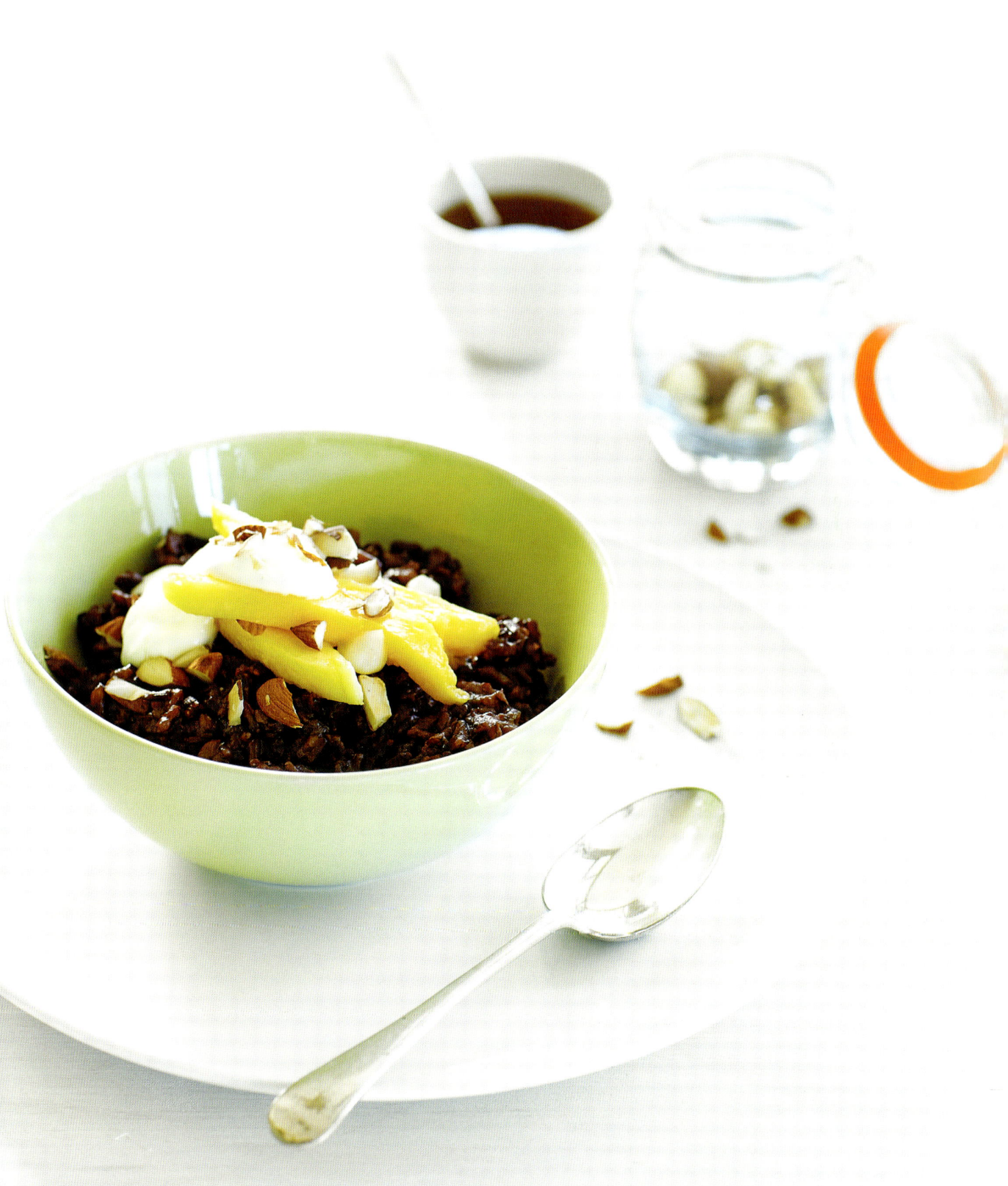

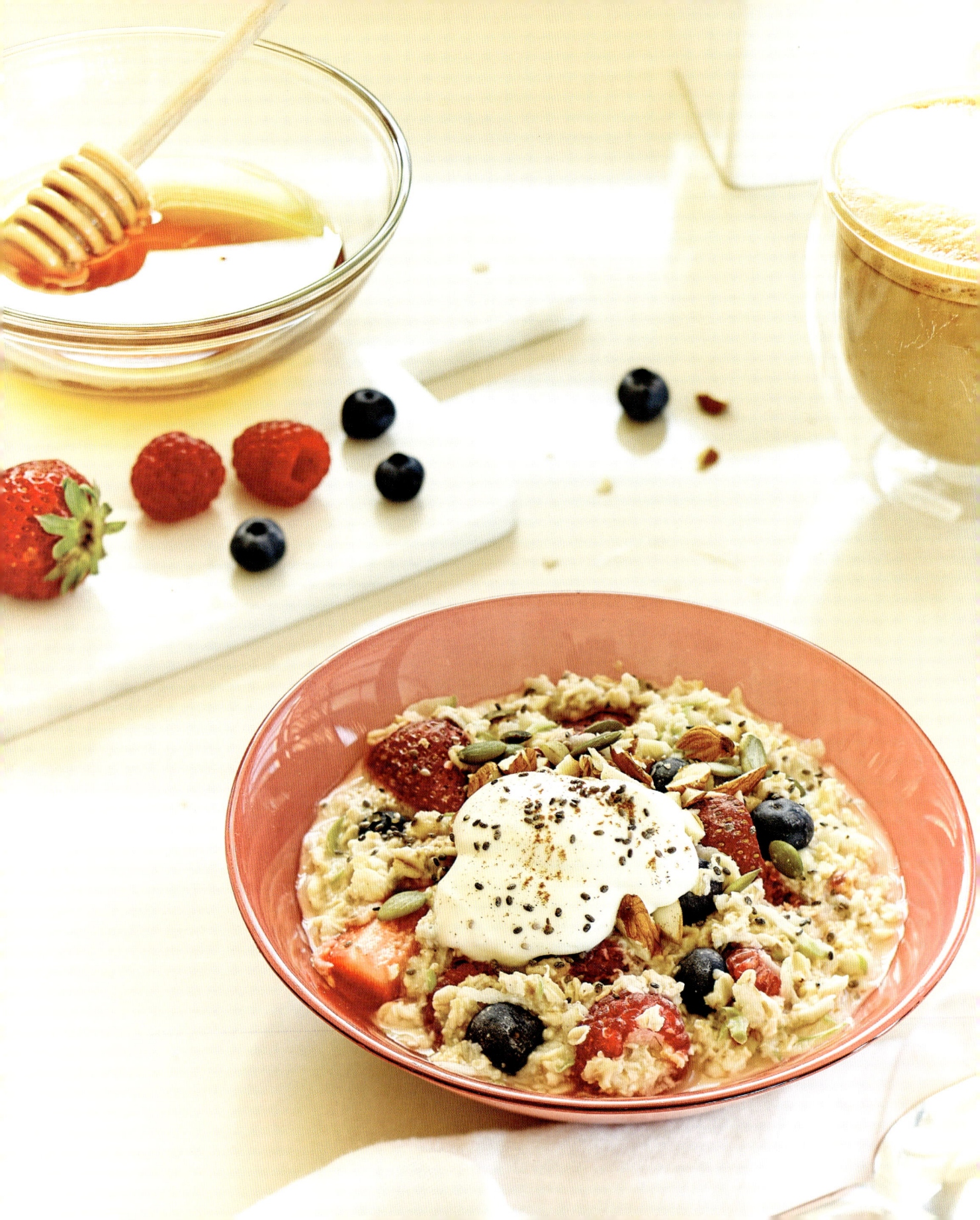

Berry Bircher Muesli
Serves 4–6

This is a great pre-made breakfast for those busy mornings when you want something nourishing as well as quick for breakfast. It lasts in the fridge for 4–5 days in an airtight container.

The chia seeds in this breakfast provide hormone regulating effects for women of all reproductive ages, as well as peri and post-menopausal women.

INGREDIENTS
200 g (7 oz) whole rolled oats
Juice of ½ lemon
2 apples with skin on, grated
375 ml (12 fl oz) water
230 g (11½ oz) frozen berries
4 tablespoons black chia seeds

Topping
20 g (1 oz) of raw nuts – almonds, brazil or walnuts, chopped
1 tablespoon pepitas or pumpkin seeds
1 teaspoon honey or maple syrup
½ teaspoon cinnamon powder
2 tablespoons natural unsweetened organic yogurt

1. The night before, mix the oats, lemon juice, water, chia, berries and apple together in a bowl. If you like your bircher sloppy, you can add more water. Cover and soak overnight.
2. In the morning, spoon a portion into your breakfast bowl and top with all or some of the toppings.

·Porridge Three Ways· *Serves 1*

Chai Tea Porridge · Coconut, Oat and Black Rice Porridge · Amaranth, Oat and Mushroom Porridge

Oats are an optimal source of B vitamins for energy and are high in soluble fiber. The fiber becomes slippery in your gut, which is a good thing. This slows the digesting time through your stomach, which makes you feel fuller longer and delays glucose absorption. This means you avoid a sugar spike in your blood. It also helps prevent constipation by softening the stool as it travels through your gut. Oats do more than this. They also contain insoluble fiber which speeds up bowel transit time through your gut and thus helps prevent constipation, plus it bulks out your stools and encourages the excretion of oestrogen.

Nut pulp: If you have some, from making nut milk, then add in a dessert spoon during cooking of any of these porridge recipes.

INGREDIENTS

- 250 ml (8 fl oz) milk (any type you like) or water
- 1 Chai teabag or loose leaf equivalent put into a personal tea infuser, or ½ teaspoon chai tea spices – star anise, cardamom, cloves, cinnamon, put into a personal tea infuser
- 45 g (2 oz) whole rolled oats
- 1 teaspoon organic butter
- Pinch of salt
- 1 tablespoon flaxseed (linseed), freshly ground
- 2–3 tablespoons unsweetened natural yogurt (any organic milk type)
- 1 handful berries, fresh or frozen
- 4 brazil nuts
- 1 tablespoon pepitas
- Cinnamon powder

1. Put the water or milk and chai tea into a saucepan and warm on the stove. Leave to infuse for about 5 minutes, then take the tea out.
2. Add the oats, butter, and salt. Turn the heat to high and bring to the boil, then turn to low and simmer for about 4 minutes until the porridge is thick and creamy. Stir regularly to stop the porridge catching on the bottom of the saucepan.
3. Pour into a breakfast bowl and stir through the ground flaxseed. This can make the porridge go thick, so add more milk if you wish.
4. Top with yogurt, berries (stir into the hot porridge if frozen), brazil nuts, pepitas and a sprinkling of cinnamon.

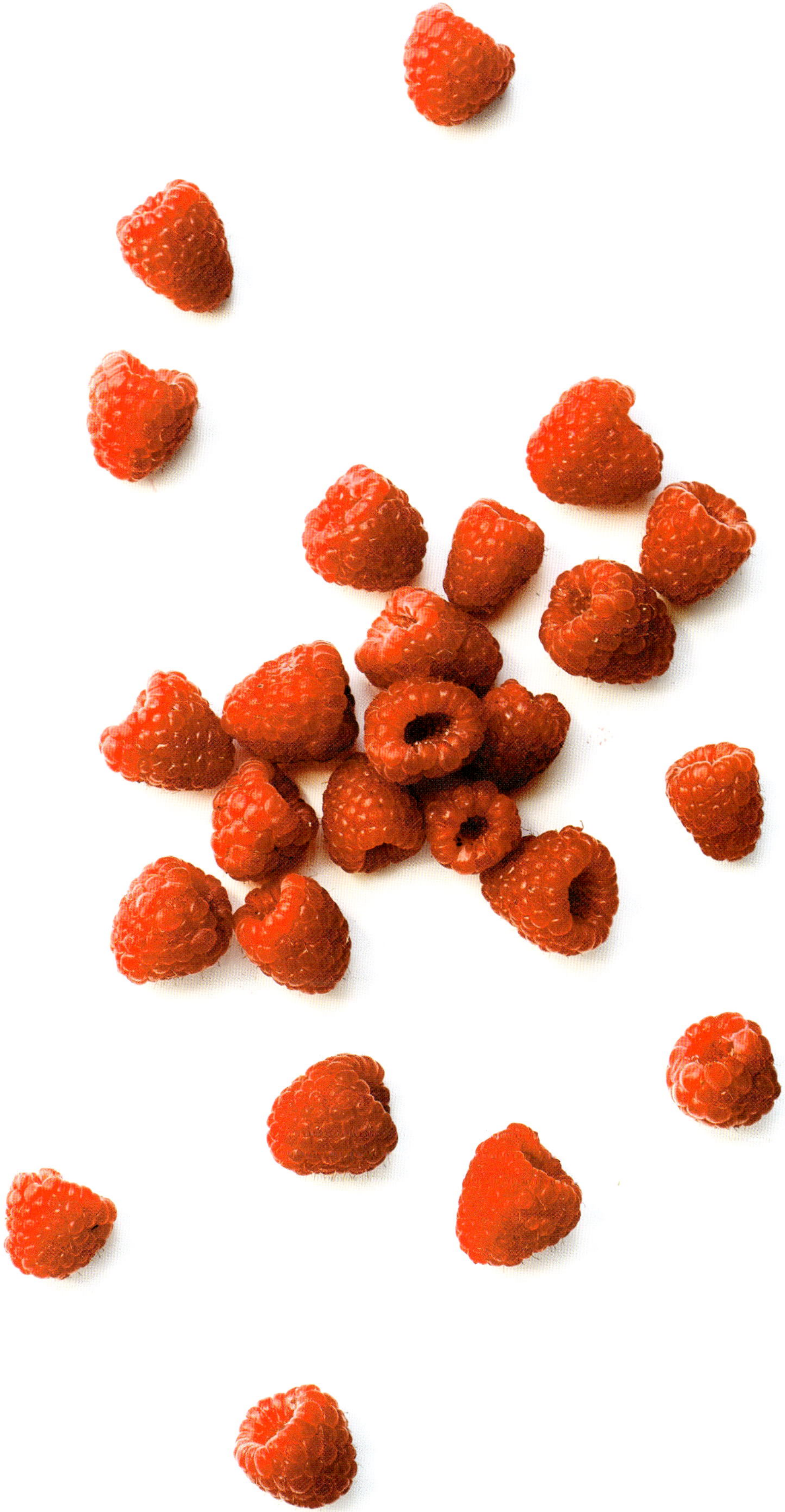

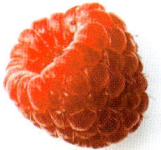

Coconut, Oat and Black Rice Porridge *Serves 1*

This breakfast bowl is fast if you already have pre-cooked black rice in your fridge or freezer. Otherwise you will need to cook the black rice first, which takes about 1 hour, following the packet instruction.

INGREDIENTS
- 40 g (2 oz) whole rolled oats
- Pinch of salt
- 1 heaped tablespoon cooked black rice
- 1 teaspoon coconut oil
- 250 ml (8 fl oz) milk (any type) or water
- 1 tablespoon black chia seeds
- 1 tablespoon coconut milk
- 2–3 tablespoons unsweetened natural organic yogurt (any type)
- 4 Brazil nuts, roughly chopped
- 1 tablespoon pepita seeds
- ½ fresh mango, skin removed, and sliced

Optional
- 1 teaspoon of honey, pure maple syrup or organic brown rice syrup
- 1 tablespoon cacao nibs

1. In a saucepan, bring to the boil the oats, salt, cooked rice, coconut oil and milk/water. Then turn the heat down to low and simmer for about 4 minutes, stirring frequently to stop the oats from sticking to the base of the saucepan.
2. Once oats are thick and creamy, pour into a breakfast bowl. Stir through the chia seeds. Pour over the coconut milk, dollop the yogurt and scatter the brazil nuts and pepitas. Place the mango strips on top.
3. If you wish, drizzle over some honey/maple/rice syrup, and scatter the cacao nibs.

Amaranth, Oat and Mushroom Porridge

Serves 1

This is a bit like savory congee with mushrooms.

INGREDIENTS

- A few dried mushrooms (if you don't have any dried mushrooms in your home, then double the quantity of fresh)
- 45 g (2 oz) fresh large field mushrooms, roughly chopped bite sized, about half a handful
- 40 g (2 oz) whole rolled oats
- 1 heaped tablespoon uncooked amaranth
- 400 ml (14 fl oz) home made vegetable, chicken or beef stock or water with 1 teaspoon miso paste
- Pinch salt
- 1 teaspoon organic butter
- 1 tablespoon sunflower seeds
- 1 tablespoon crumbled goat or sheep feta
- 1 heaped teaspoon fresh chopped parsley or thyme or rosemary
- A pinch freshly ground black pepper

1. Wash the dried mushrooms. Place them with the oats, amaranth and broth/water into a saucepan and soak for about 10 minutes, whilst you get everything else ready.
2. Add salt, butter and fresh mushrooms, then cook with the oats, amaranth, broth/water and dried mushrooms on high heat. Bring to the boil, then turn the heat down to low and simmer until the oats are soft and the amaranth is cooked, about 10 minutes. Stir frequently to stop the oats from sticking to the base of the pan.
3. Pour into your breakfast bowl and sprinkle with sunflower seeds, feta and parsley.

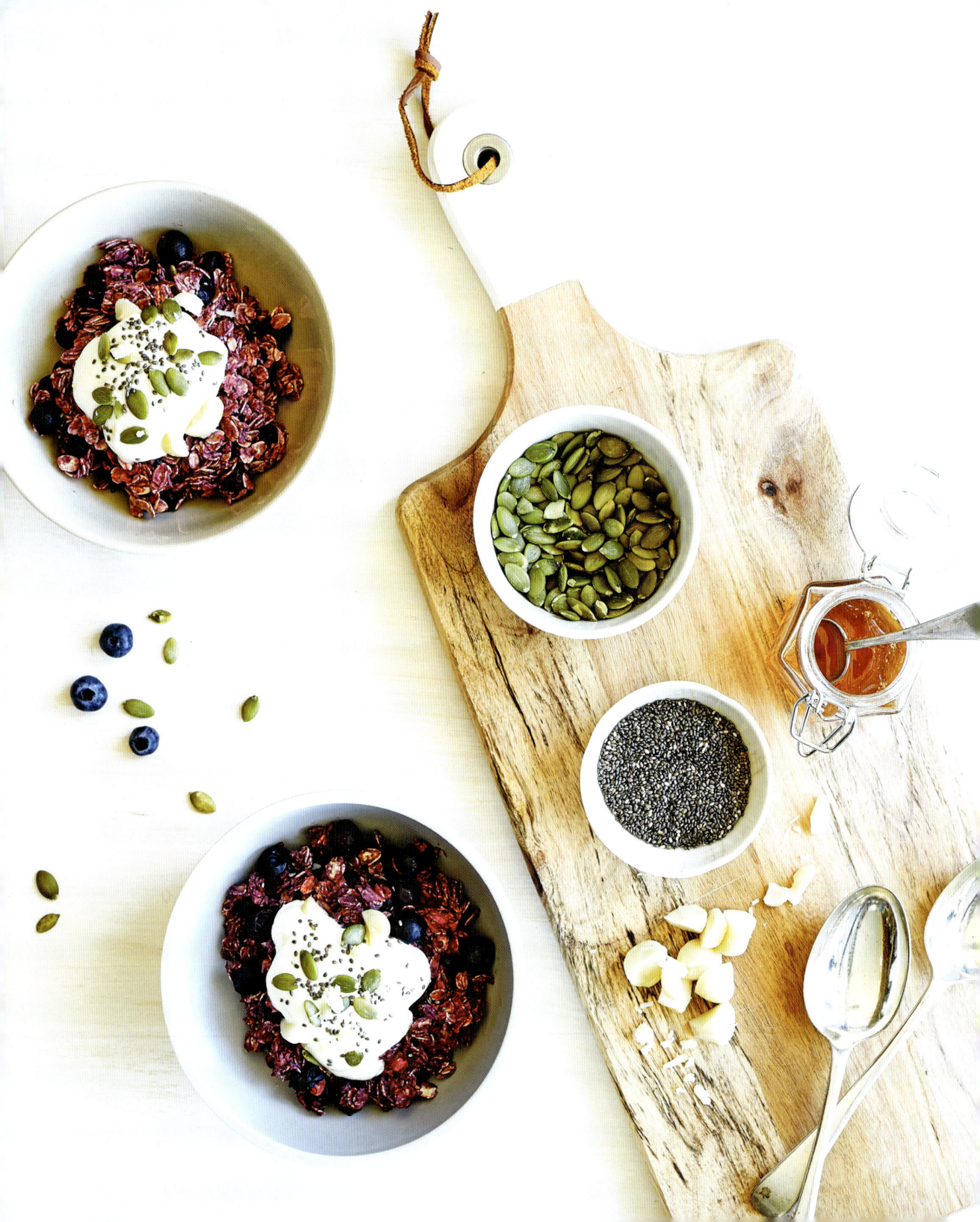

•Pink Oats• *Serves 1*

Fast, smart, and pretty! These Pink Oats are a great choice because they contain:
- anthocyanin (colorful) flavonoid antioxidants from the berries
- fiber from the oats and chia seeds
- anti-inflammatory oils from the nuts and seeds

The pumpkin seeds provide the precursor amino acid Tryptophan which is used in the biosynthesis of serotonin, the 'happy-mood enhancing' neurotransmitter.

INGREDIENTS
115 g (4 oz) mixed berries (fresh or frozen). Emma likes blueberry and blackcurrants mixed
27 g (1 oz) whole rolled oats
1 tablespoon black chia seeds
1 tablespoon pumpkin seeds
20 g (1 oz) macadamia nuts, chopped
2 heaped tablespoons natural unsweetened organic yogurt
Acai powder, optional

1. In a breakfast bowl, mash the berries with the oats and chia seeds. Spoon the yogurt into the bowl and mix through, making the oats pink. Sprinkle the chopped nuts and seeds over the top. Add the Acai powder, if you wish. Then it really is a pink start to the day.

Jill's Digestive Muesli

Makes 10 serves and lasts up to 5 weeks, when stored in the fridge

High in fiber, this muesli aids liver clearance of excess oestrogens and helps bowel function. The minerals in the nuts and seeds support hormone production and your liver's detoxification functions. The phytoestrogens in the nuts, seeds and wholegrains help reduce symptoms of menopause and menstrual problems.

INGREDIENTS

- 70 g (3 oz) pepitas
- 70 g (3 oz) sunflower seeds
- 70 g (3 oz) flaxseed (linseed) meal (requires refrigeration)
- 70 g (3 oz) sesame seeds
- 70 g (3 oz) roasted almonds, chopped
- 70 g (3 oz) naturally dried fruit (not cranberries due to their high sugar content)
- 70 g (3 oz) oat bran
- 70 g (3 oz) lecithin granules (requires refrigeration)
- 70 g (3 oz) black chia seeds
- 150 g (5 oz) rice bran cereal
- 200 g (7 oz) organic rolled oats

1. In a large bowl, thoroughly mix all ingredients together. Spoon into an airtight glass container and store in the fridge to ensure it retains the nutrients, especially of the flaxseed (linseed) meal and lecithin granules.

   Note: 100 g (3 oz) is an ideal and sustaining breakfast each day. Jill serves this with rice milk, coconut or organic yogurt and fresh or frozen blueberries.

Lentil Cakes with Poached Eggs
Serves 2

Broad beans and lentils provide a great source of isoflavones – plant derived compounds with oestrogenic activity – helping to potentially balance both high and low oestrogen.

Spinach is great source of:
- anti-inflammatory phytonutrients, especially for the gut
- Vitamin K and calcium for bone health
- Carotenoids for ovarian health
- Magnesium for neurological and bone health
- Vitamin C, a cofactor in the production of dopamine, the 'zest for life' neurotransmitter

INGREDIENTS
- 2 small potatoes, wash and leave skin on
- 1 teaspoon ground cumin
- 2 tablespoons extra virgin olive oil or organic butter
- 2 tablespoons broad beans (fava beans) shelled, lightly cooked or defrosted if frozen
- 75 g (3 oz) cooked red lentils (cook your own or canned), lightly smashed
- 1 small garlic clove, crushed
- 4 organic free range eggs
- 2 big handfuls washed spinach leaves
- Salt and freshly ground black pepper

1. Grate the potatoes. Toss them with the cumin powder and gently cook in a frying pan with 1 tablespoon of butter/oil until softening. The potato should be sticky and glue like. Set aside to cool.
2. Using your hands, mix the broad beans, lentils, garlic, potato, salt and pepper together in a bowl. Firmly shape the mixture into cakes. Fry them on medium heat, in the remaining tablespoon of butter/oil, until crisp on both sides.
3. Whilst the lentil cakes are cooking, poach the eggs in simmering water for 3–4 minutes, aiming to keep the yolk soft.
4. Finish by wilting the spinach leaves in the frying pan, once the lentil cakes are cooked. Add the salt and pepper. This should take 1–2 minutes.
5. Divide the lentil cakes between 2 serving plates. Add the spinach and top with the eggs.

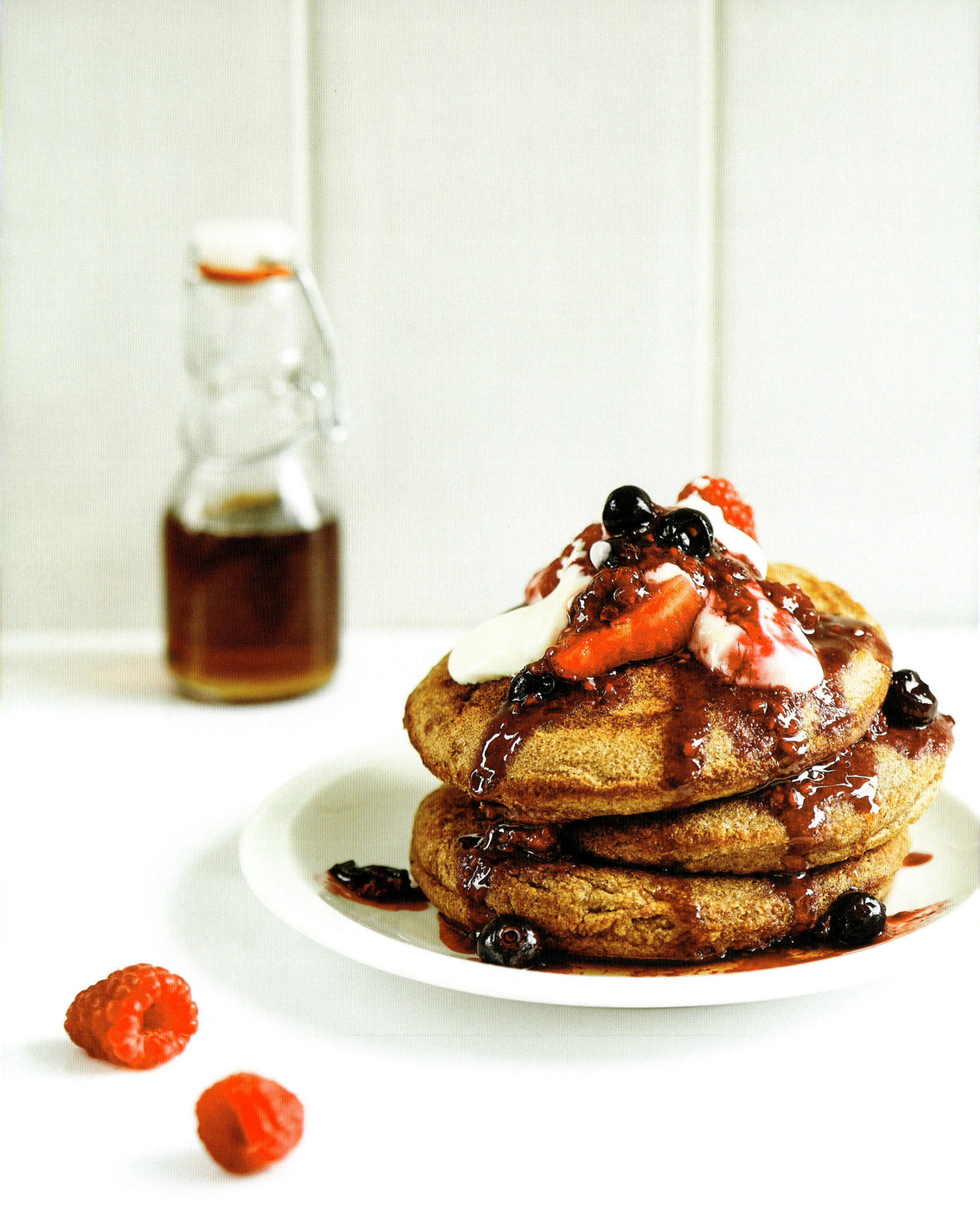

Buckwheat Pancakes with Smashed Berries

Serves 1 / Makes 2 pancakes

The flaxseeds in these delicious pancakes are a rich source of dietary fiber, good oils, lignans and isoflavones. These provide soothing soluble dietary fiber, anti-inflammatory essential fatty acids, modulate oestrogen and help to reduce oestrogen reabsorption from the bowel. The cinnamon, apart from a great flavor, helps with your blood glucose balance.

INGREDIENTS

- 1 egg, beaten
- 100 ml (3 fl oz) milk (almond, rice, oat, soy, organic cow)
- 1 tablespoon melted organic butter, plus 1 teaspoon for the pan
- 25 g (1 oz) buckwheat flour (or whole wheat flour)
- 1 tablespoon flaxseed (linseed), freshly ground
- ½ teaspoon baking powder
- 1 teaspoon cinnamon powder
- 1 teaspoon 100 per cent maple syrup, honey or brown rice syrup
- 1 heaped tablespoon nut pulp (if you have it from making nut milk)
- 1 large handful washed fresh or frozen berries
- 3 tablespoons natural unsweetened yogurt (organic cow's, goat, sheep, buffalo or coconut)

1. Mix all the ingredients, except for the berries and yogurt, together in a bowl using a fork or whisk.
2. Heat a small frying pan/skillet on low. This is to ensure the pancakes don't burn before you flip them and the delicate flaxseed oils don't over heat.
3. Brush the pan with 1 teaspoon of butter.
4. Pour in half the mixture and cook on one side for about one minute. Then flip and cook on the other side for about 40 seconds or until the pancake is just cooked through to the center. Repeat with the second pancake.
5. Mash up the berries. Once both pancakes are cooked, put them onto a serving plate and pile the berries on top. Add the yogurt and, if you wish, drizzle a little maple syrup over the top.

Note: In particular use blueberries, blackcurrants and blackberries, as these are highest in phytonutrients.

Apple and Cinnamon Flapjacks

Serves 4 – 6

Once made, these flapjacks provide a fast portable breakfast or snack.

When grains, such as whole rolled oats, are eaten in their whole form, they retain their powerful phytonutrients. Oats and apples also contain soluble and insoluble fiber (see Porridge page 42), which has been shown to increase the body's elimination of oestrogens and may reduce circulating oestrogen levels.

INGREDIENTS

- 2 large apples
- 4 tablespoons water
- 1–2 tablespoons maple syrup, honey or brown rice syrup
- 3 tablespoons extra virgin olive oil
- 2 tablespoons almond butter or quality peanut butter
- 2 teaspoons cinnamon powder
- 170 g (6 oz) whole rolled oats
- 1 heaped tablespoon black chia seeds
- 70 g (3 oz) pumpkin seeds
- 70 g (3 oz) raw almonds, roughly chopped
- 40 g (2 oz) dried currants or sultanas, sulfur-dioxide free
- Pinch of salt

1. Set your oven to 180°C (350°F) fan forced or 200°C (400°F) regular oven.
2. Wash and core the apples, then grate them, with their skins left on, into a medium sized saucepan.
3. Add 4 tablespoons of water and cook on low-medium heat until the apple softens (about 15 minutes). Stir occasionally and keep the lid on when not stirring. The apples are cooked once they become soft and sauce-like.
4. In a mixing bowl add the maple syrup, olive oil, nut butter and cinnamon. Mix together well.
5. Once cooked, add the apple mixture and roughly combine. Then add the oats, seeds, nuts and salt and roughly mix.
6. Line a brownie pan 20 cm x 20 cm (8 inch x 8 inch) with baking/parchment paper and pour in the oat mixture. Press down firmly to spread the mixture evenly across the pan, then flatten the top.
7. Bake for 25 minutes or until the top of the flapjacks looks slightly browned.
8. Take out of the oven and leave in the pan to cool to room temperature. They will become crisp.
9. Carefully tip out onto a board and cut into portions. If you wish to crisp them further, put the pieces back in the oven on a baking tray for 5–10 minutes.

Note: Quality peanut butter is one that is made from peanuts with no added oils or sugar.

Overnight Berry Oats
Serves 1

There's everything nutritious in this breakfast. Soluble fiber in the oats, chia and flaxseeds assist your liver to do its job, especially with excreting excess oestrogen. There is a high anthocyanin phytonutrient content in the berries and high mineral content in the nuts and seeds. These all help with female hormone balance. The beneficial gut bacteria in the yogurt helps your gut to function well and absorb nutrients.

INGREDIENTS

- 40 g (1½ oz) whole rolled oats
- 1 tablespoon black chia seeds
- 120 ml (4 fl oz) water or any type of milk
- 100 g (3½ oz) blueberries (fresh or frozen)
- 50 g (2 oz) raspberries (fresh or frozen)
- 2 heaped tablespoons natural unsweetened organic yogurt
- 1 tablespoon flaxseed (linseed), freshly ground
- 4 brazil nuts, roughly chopped
- 5 raw almonds, roughly chopped
- 1 teaspoon cinnamon powder
- Honey, pure maple syrup or brown rice syrup, optional

1. You will need a 500 ml (16 fl oz) open neck jam jar, ideally a mason or preserving jar.
2. Put the oats and chia seeds into the bottom. Add the water/milk and mix well.
3. Then add the blueberries and raspberries, followed by the yogurt.
4. Scatter the ground flaxseed, brazil nuts, almonds and cinnamon on top. Drizzle a little honey, maple syrup or brown rice syrup, if you like extra sweetness.
5. Leave in the fridge overnight. The oats and chia seeds will soak up the liquid. In the morning your breakfast will be ready.

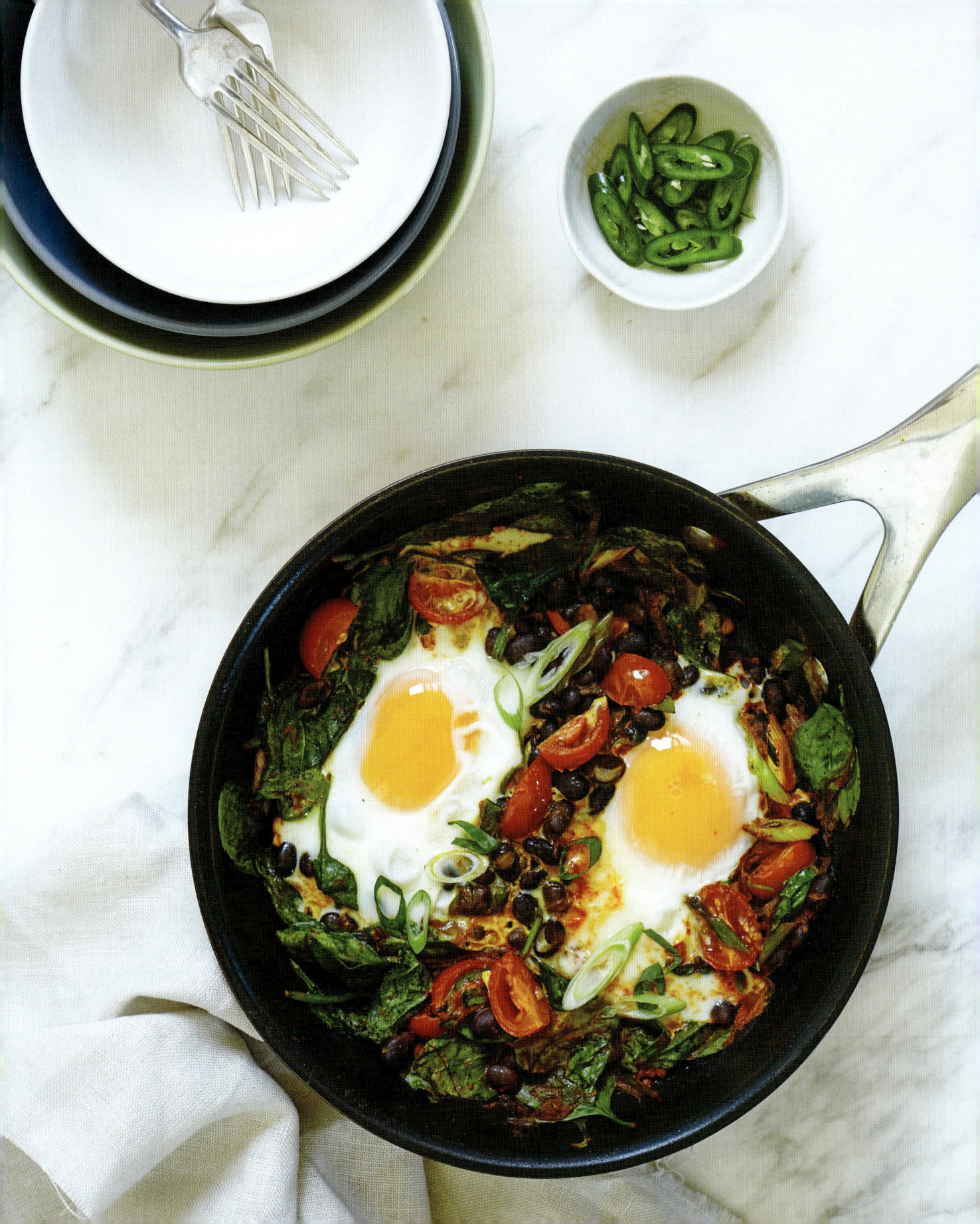

Ranch Eggs with Spinach
Serves 1

This is Emma's family's all-time favorite breakfast, which is saying something as they have a big range to choose from, having been exposed to all sorts of breakfasts over time. Often it's eaten for lunch or a fast dinner when no one else is around to share dinner with. This breakfast is high in fiber, minerals, protein, phytonutrients and taste – an all round winner.

INGREDIENTS

- 1 tablespoon extra virgin olive oil
- 1 teaspoon turmeric
- ½ teaspoon cumin seeds or powder
- 1 large spring onion (scallion), chopped (white and green parts)
- 5 cherry tomatoes, chopped
- 2 tablespoons tomato passatta (if you have it)
- 60 g (2½ oz) cooked black beans (cook your own or canned)
- 1 handful chopped spinach/chard/kale/silverbeet
- 2 organic free range eggs
- 1 heaped tablespoon natural unsweetened yogurt
- Pinch salt and pepper
- 1 teaspoon apple cider vinegar

Optional extra:
- ½ teaspoon long red chili/jalapeño chili, chopped or splash of Tabasco sauce

1. In a small frying pan/skillet set on medium heat, gently warm the olive oil and cumin seeds, about 30 seconds.
2. Add the spring onions, tomatoes, and tomato passatta (if using). Warm and slightly cook the onion and tomatoes for about a minute.
3. Add the spinach and beans. Stir to warm, then crack in the 2 eggs. Cook until the egg white is just firm, but the yolk soft, about 3 minutes. Remove the pan from the heat.
4. Dollop the yogurt on top, scatter the chopped chili and splash the vinegar over. Add salt and pepper to taste. Eat straight from the pan.

Field Mushrooms with Saffron Yogurt

Serves 1

In Traditional Chinese Medicine saffron is thought to stimulate the qi energy of the liver, remove stagnation and release toxins. It is also thought to reduce irritation and distress in menopause.

Field mushrooms are high in vitamin B5, which helps to modulate secretion of the stress hormone cortisol from your adrenal glands. It is particularly beneficial for those with a stressful busy life and/or heading into menopause. B5 is involved in the release of energy from your food.

INGREDIENTS
Small red onion, finely chopped
1 tablespoon extra virgin olive oil
½ teaspoon cumin seeds
2 large field mushrooms, thickly sliced
3 tablespoons cooked lentils
1 handful washed spinach leaves
1 teaspoon apple cider vinegar

Saffron Yogurt
2 tablespoons yogurt, natural unsweetened organic
½ small garlic clove, peeled and crushed
Pinch of saffron fronds
Salt and pepper

1. Put the extra virgin olive oil, cumin seeds and onion into a frying pan/skillet on low heat, to slowly cook. Stir occasionally until the onions begin to soften, about 3 minutes.
2. Turn the heat up to medium and toss in the mushrooms. Stir occasionally to avoid the ingredients sticking. Allow the mushrooms to cook until soft, then stir in the lentils to warm. Stir in the spinach to wilt.
3. Combine the saffron and garlic with the yogurt, saving a few fronds to decorate the top.
4. Spoon the mushroom mix into a serving bowl. Add a pinch of salt and pepper. Sprinkle the apple cider vinegar over the mushrooms and dollop the saffron yogurt on top, sprinkling some saffron fronds to finish.

Note: You can swap the lentils for cooked chickpeas. Break up the chickpeas with your spoon as you warm them in the pan.

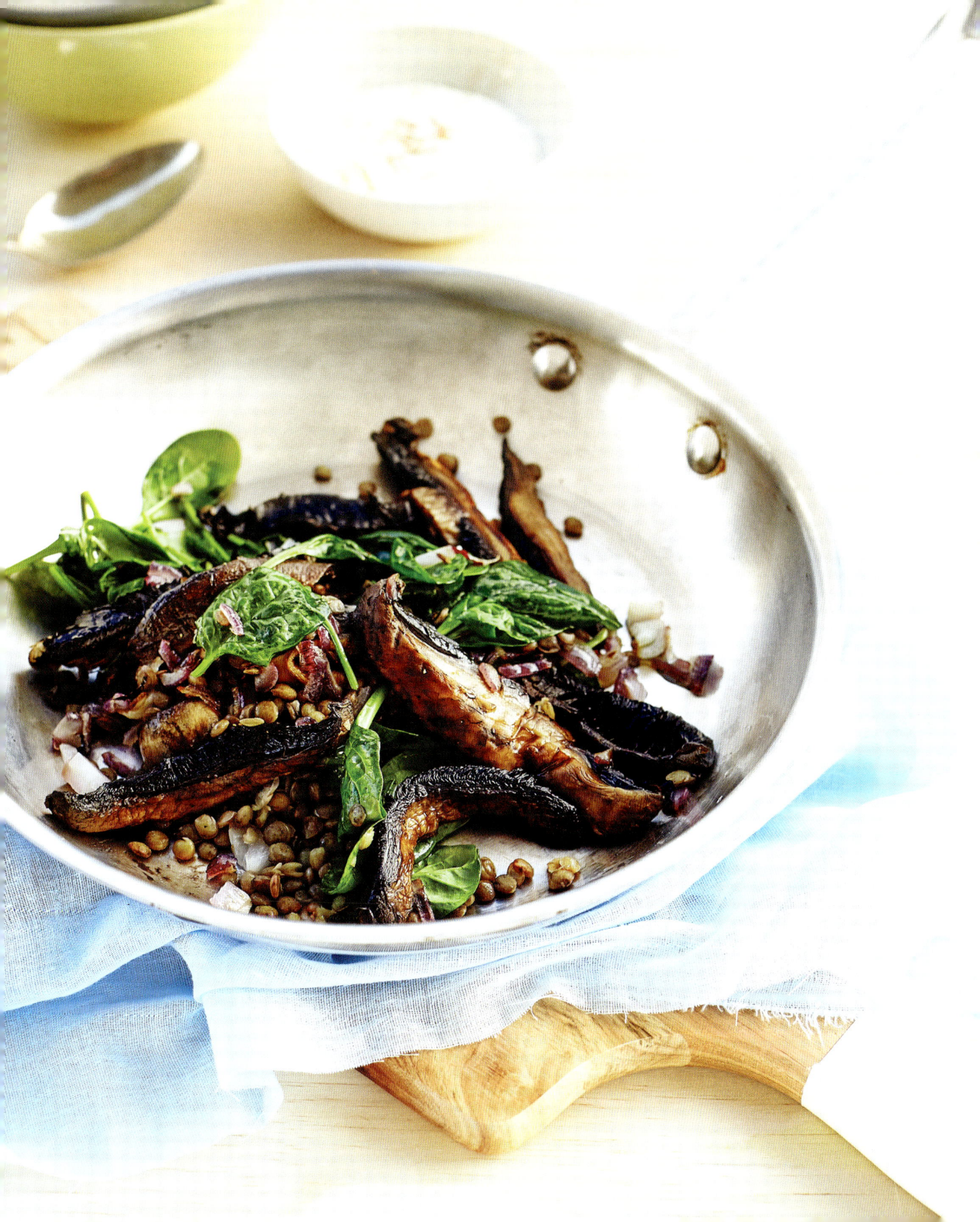

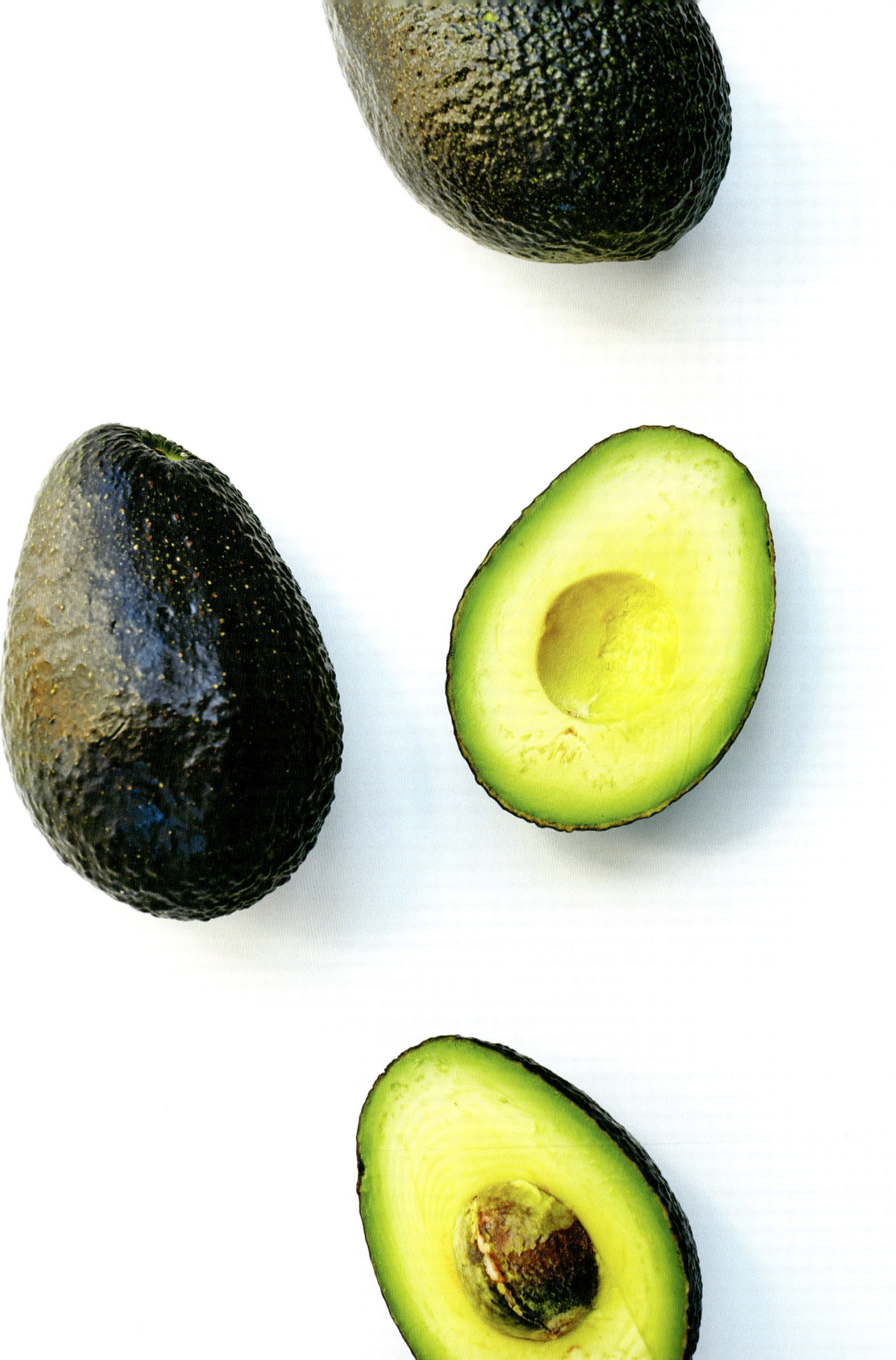

Home-Cured Salmon with Avocado
Serves 1, with leftover sauce

Omega 3 oils, found in large amounts in salmon, are highly beneficial to both menstrual and menopausal issues. They help to enhance mood and reduce inflammation throughout the body.

INGREDIENTS
50 g (1 oz) home-cured salmon (see recipe page 32), sliced or smoked salmon

Avocado smash
½ large avocado
½ tablespoon lemon juice
1 tablespoon flaxseed (linseed), freshly ground
Pinch salt and freshly ground pepper

Sauce
1 teaspoon Dijon mustard
1 teaspoon horseradish sauce (with a minimum 60 per cent horseradish content) or freshly grated horseradish root
1 tablespoon unsweetened natural organic yogurt (goat, sheep, organic cow, buffalo)
Pinch of salt and freshly ground pepper
1 teaspoon apple cider vinegar
1 teaspoon honey

1. In a bowl, using a fork, smash and mix the avocado with lemon juice, ground flaxseed and salt and pepper. Place onto your serving plate.
2. Mix the mustard, horseradish, yogurt, salt, pepper, vinegar and honey together in a small bowl.
3. Place the sliced salmon on top of the smash and add a heaped tablespoon of the sauce.
4. This is delicious with rye bread toast or gluten-free buckwheat toast. Spread the smash on.

Note: If you are not eating bread, you can add a small handful of lentil sprouts or 2 tablespoons of cooked lentils to the smash, if you wish.

Spanish-style Tortilla with Mushrooms

Serves 1

This is a fast, easy to make breakfast. Mushrooms are an excellent source of fiber (along with the chickpeas), as well as B vitamins. These are used in the body for energy production, liver detoxification and for hormone balance for women who are menopausal or experience PMS. Parsley is high in ovary-loving vitamin C and acts as a diuretic, which aids the clearance of fluid for women with PMS. Along with chickpeas, it also helps provide isoflavones which act as phytoestrogens, helping to balance oestrogen.

INGREDIENTS
- 1 tablespoon extra virgin olive oil
- 1 spring onion (scallion), washed and finely chopped
- ¼ long green or jalapeño chili, deseeded and finely chopped
- 1 large field mushroom, sliced
- 1 handful parsley leaves, washed and finely chopped
- 1 tablespoon cooked chickpeas, lightly smashed
- Big pinch of salt and freshly ground pepper
- 2 tablespoons freshly grated Parmesan or Pecorino cheese, optional
- 2 large organic free range eggs
- ½ teaspoon apple cider vinegar

1. In a small frying pan/skillet, on medium heat, fry the oil, onion, chili and mushrooms. Toss until the mushrooms are just soft, about 4 minutes.
2. Add the parsley, chickpeas, salt, pepper, cheese and crack in the eggs. Swirl together a little. Then put a lid on the pan and cook for 1–2 minutes, until the whites are just firm. This will cook quickly, as the vegetables are already hot.
3. Drizzle the apple cider vinegar on top. Eat straight out of the pan or slide onto a plate and enjoy.

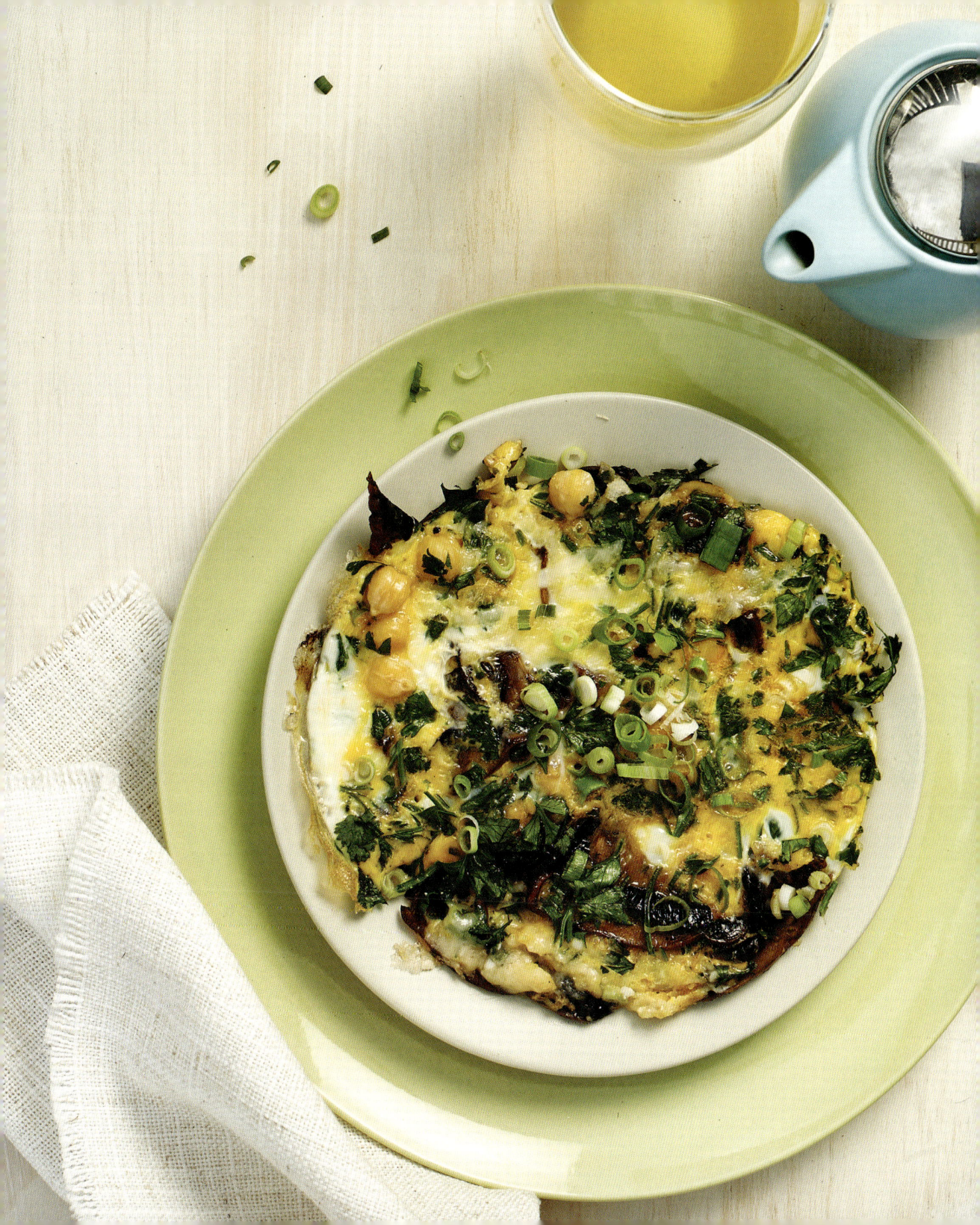

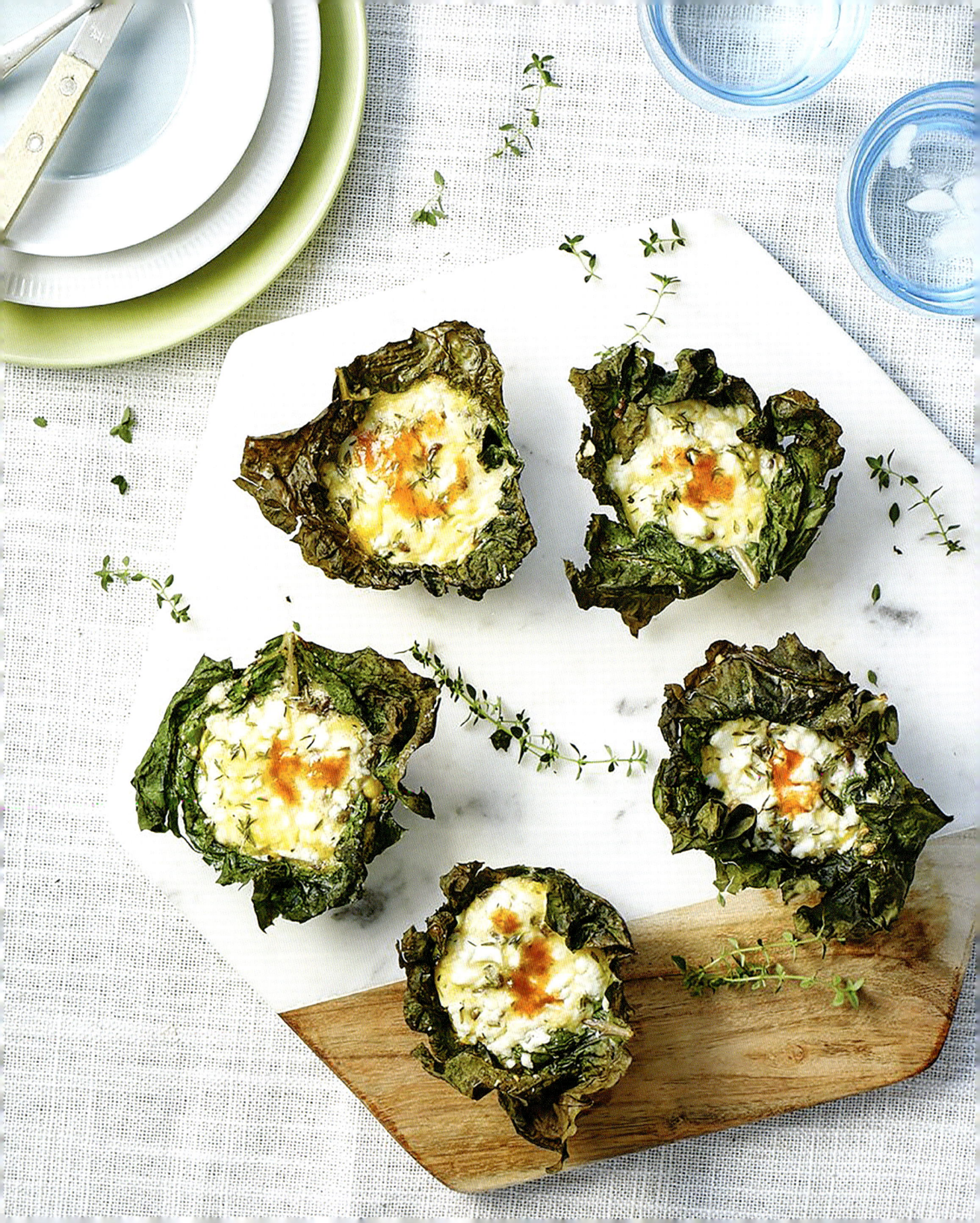

Green Egg Pies

Serves 1 / Makes 2 pies

These pies offer good fiber from the lentils to help clear out excess oestrogens. The vitamin C and magnesium from the spinach help combat the effects of stress. Eggs provide a good source of protein, as well as B group vitamins (along with the spinach) needed for neurotransmitter (good mood hormone) production.

INGREDIENTS

- 1 tablespoon extra virgin olive oil
- 2 large spinach, silverbeet or chard leaves, about 12 cm x 12 cm (4.5 inch x 4.5 inch), washed and dried
- Big pinch of salt and freshly ground pepper
- 2 large organic free range eggs
- 2 tablespoons cooked lentils
- 1 heaped teaspoon fresh chopped rosemary or thyme leaves
- 1 heaped tablespoon crumbled goat or sheep feta
- A dash of chili sauce, optional

1. Heat the oven to 180°C (350°F) fan forced or 200°C (390°F) regular.
2. Lightly oil 2 muffin holes in a regular sized muffin pan or 125 ml (4 fl oz) ovenproof pots.
3. Brush a little oil onto the leaves, then fit them snugly into the muffin tins, with some of the leaf coming up out of the hole. It is important there are no holes, tears or gaps in your leaf as the egg mixture will seep through and stick to the pots.
4. Lightly sprinkle salt and pepper onto the leaves.
5. Crack the eggs into a bowl. Add the lentils, rosemary, feta and a pinch of salt and pepper. Using a fork, lightly mix together so that the egg is not fully blended.
6. Divide the egg mixture between the two pots.
7. Bake in the oven for 15 minutes, until only just set. Remove and splash a dash of chili sauce over the top.
8. Allow to cool for 5–10 minutes before eating

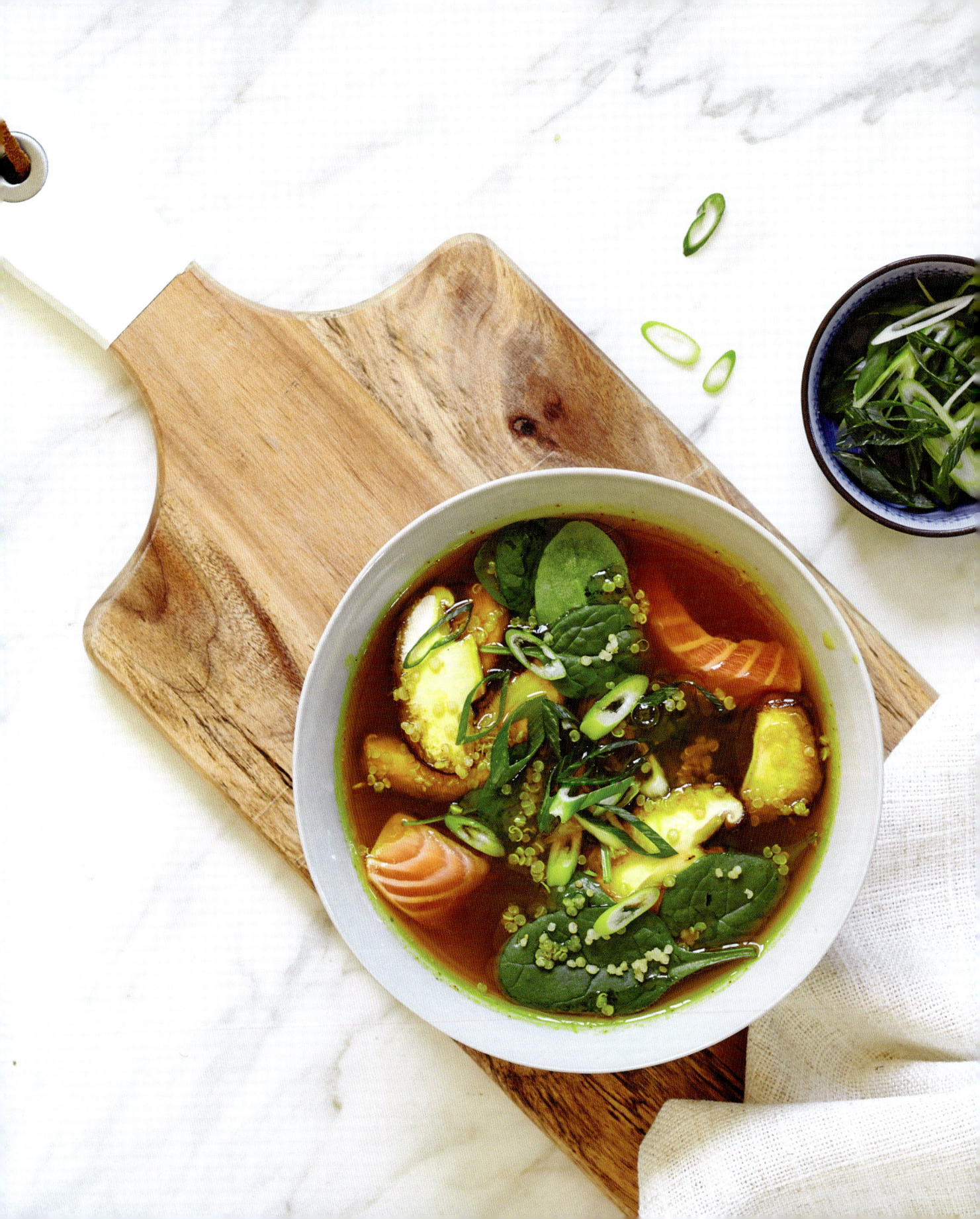

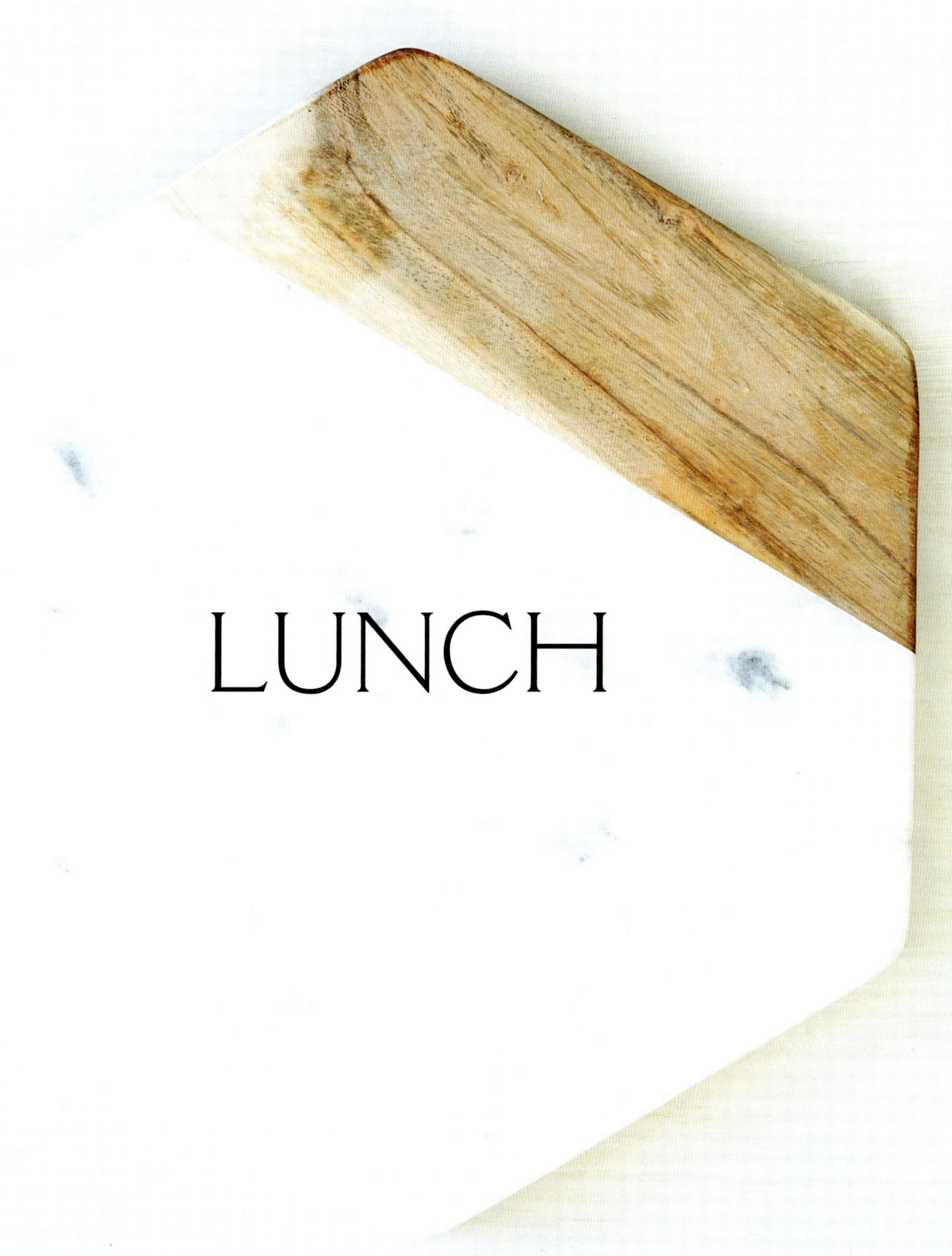

LUNCH

Salad in a Jar (V) *Serves 1*

This is the perfect on-the-move lunch. We find the best salads have some leftover vegetables, such as roasted beetroot and cauliflower, plus the staple salads you have in the fridge. You can make any combination you want, using your preferred quantities. Make sure you add some vibrant greens and brassica vegetables because they help alleviate symptoms of elevated oestrogen such as PMS, acne, weight gain and annoying menopausal symptoms. Add in sprouted pulses for phytoestrogens and fiber.

Brassica vegetables include cauliflower, brussel sprouts, cabbage including Chinese cabbage (wombok), broccoli/broccolini, watercress, radishes and green leafy vegetables such as bok choy, rocket (arugula), collard greens and kale.

This salad is easy to throw together and helps keep your hormones happy!

INGREDIENTS

Salad dressing
2 tablespoons extra virgin olive oil
1 tablespoon fresh lemon juice
1 teaspoon tahini
Big pinch of salt and pepper

Salad
3 florets of roasted cauliflower
3 pieces of roasted beetroot
3 green beans, blanched and chopped
½ carrot, peeled and coarsely grated
1 tablespoon sprouted lentils
100 g (3½ oz) organic silken tofu
1 sprig of fresh mint, chopped
½ handful baby spinach, washed
25 g (1 oz) chickpeas, cooked
½ tablespoon pickled ginger (see recipe page 35)

1. You will need a 500 ml (16 fl oz) mason or similar glass jar with a wide opening.
2. Pour the olive oil, tahini and lemon juice into the jar. Add the salt and pepper. Mix the dressing with a fork. Then layer each of the salad ingredients in the order listed above in the jar.
3. Seal the jar and keep in the fridge until you are ready to eat it. Remove from the fridge. Tip the jar upside down and shake the dressing through the salad. Either eat from the jar or pour onto a serving plate.

Note: If refrigerating for later use, it is best to place the firmer vegetables on top of the dressing, so that the salad leaves don't go soggy.

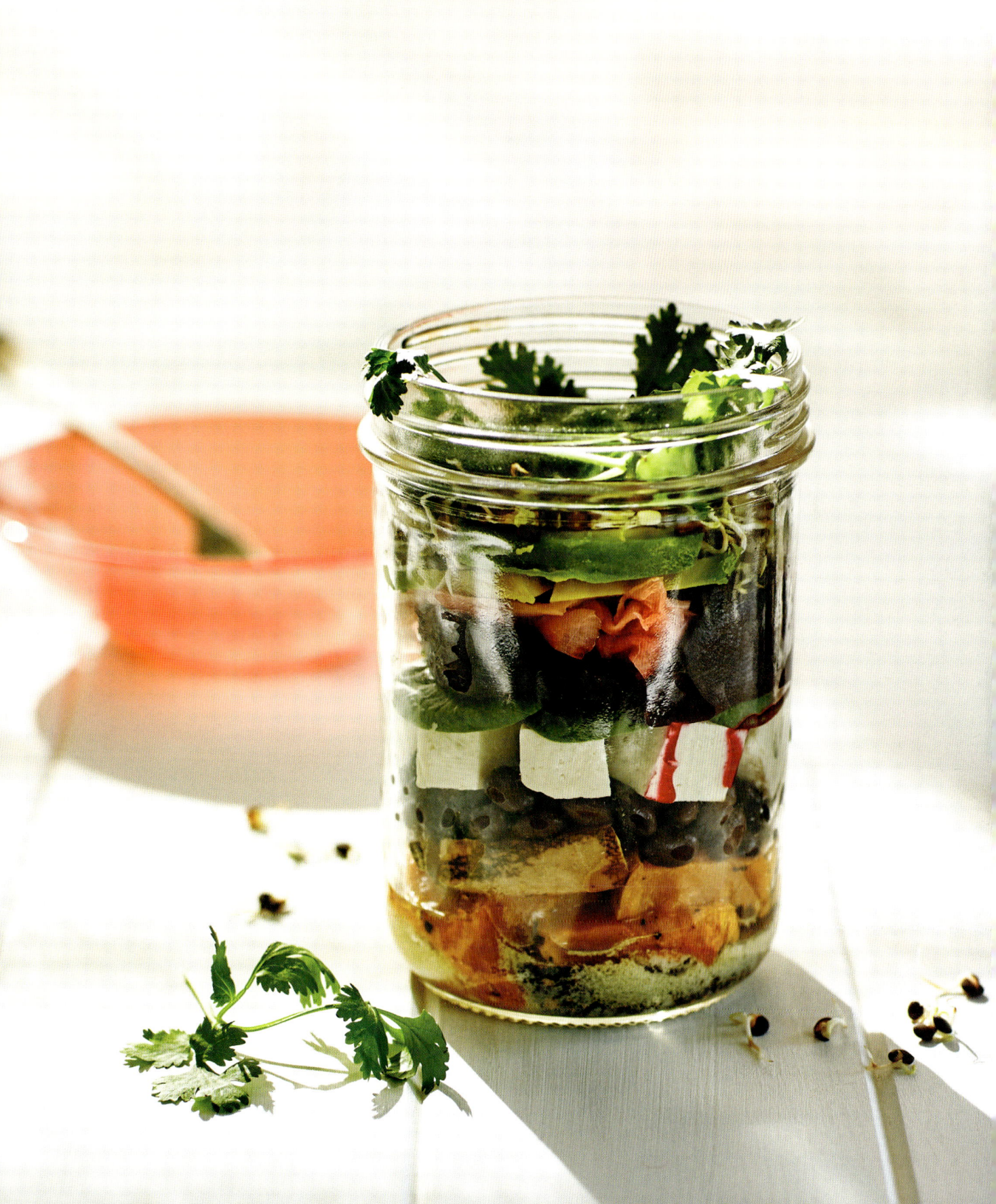

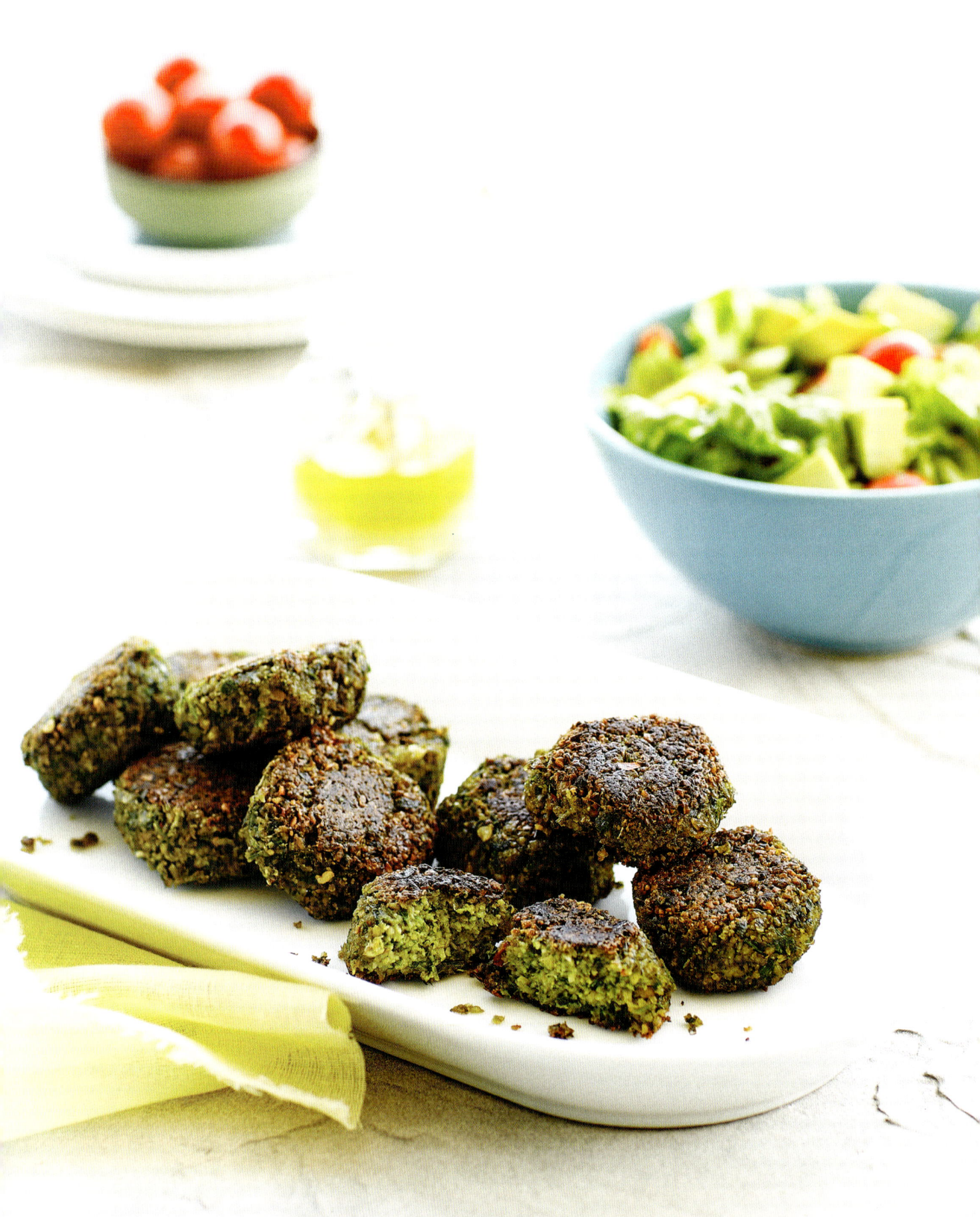

Falafels with Avocado and Oregano Salad (V)

Makes about 15 falafels / Salad serves 2 with leftover falafels

Falafels contain plenty of beneficial phytoestrogens, which help to balance oestrogen. Lentils and broad beans (fava beans) provide natural fiber to help clear and prevent oestrogen reabsorption. They are also a good source of bone-building calcium. The healthy fats in the avocado and extra virgin olive oil, help to reduce inflammation and support hormone balance.

INGREDIENTS

Falafels
- 200 g (7 oz) dried skinless split broad beans/fava beans, soaked overnight in water. Yields about 300 g (7½ oz) soaked beans.
- 2 handfuls fresh coriander (cilantro) leaves, washed
- 2 handfuls fresh continental (flat leaf) parsley leaves, washed
- 60 g (2½ oz) spring onions (scallions), roughly chopped (white and green parts)
- 3 large garlic cloves, peeled and crushed
- 2 teaspoons ground cumin
- 2 teaspoons ground coriander
- 1 teaspoon salt
- Big pinch cayenne pepper
- Big pinch ground ginger
- 1 teaspoon baking powder (aluminum and gluten-free)
- 100 g (3½ oz) cooked chickpeas
- Extra virgin olive oil

Salad
- ½ large ripe avocado, de-seeded, skinned and roughly chopped
- Heart of 1 cos lettuce, chopped (about 2 handfuls)
- 100 g (3½ oz) cherry tomatoes, washed and quartered
- 1 small Lebanese cucumber, washed and chopped
- 1 large lemon, juiced
- 4 tablespoons extra virgin olive oil
- 2 teaspoons dried Greek oregano
- 1 heaped tablespoon goat feta, crumbled
- 2 heaped tablespoons hummus (recipe page 184)

To make falafels:
1. Drain the broad beans and put into a food processor with all other falafel ingredients except for the chickpeas and olive oil. Blend until well combined and the broad beans have broken down into a coarse pulp.
2. Scrape down the sides of your processor bowl and blend again until all is well mixed.
3. Add the chickpeas and blend until they have just broken up but have not gone to a pulp. Let the mixture rest for about half an hour.
4. Wash your hands and dry them. Scoop a tablespoon of the mixture into your hand and roll into a small ball. Repeat until you have used all the mixture.
5. Warm a large frying pan/skillet on medium heat, add the olive oil to shallow fry the falafels, so the oil is only half way up the sides of the falafel.
6. Once you have put them into the pan, gently flatten them so they are disk shaped. Cook for 2–3 minutes on one side, then turn over and cook for 2–3 minutes on the other. Depending on the size of your pan, you may have to cook them in batches.

To make salad:
1. Toss all the salad ingredients, except for the hummus, together in a salad bowl. Divide the salad between two plates, scatter the feta over the top, and place 3 or 4 falafels on top plus a dollop of hummus.

·All-Things-Green Warming Broth· Serves 1

A fast, easy broth that's so delicious, yet so simple to make. Green vegetables tend to be high in B vitamins, which are used in our bodies to create energy, renew cells and for 'good mood' hormone production.

INGREDIENTS

- 1 spring onion (scallion), white and green parts finely chopped
- 1 tablespoon extra virgin olive oil
- 300 ml (10 fl oz) homemade vegetable, chicken or beef broth
- ½ zucchini (courgette), grated
- 40 g (½ oz) cooked pulses such as green lentils, or chickpeas (cook your own or canned)
- 1 big handful green leaves – spinach, kale, silverbeet, chard or tuscan cabbage, whatever you have, washed and roughly chopped
- 2 teaspoons homemade parsley oil (recipe page 75)
- 20 g (1 oz) freshly grated Parmesan or Manchego cheese or a smoked hard cheese, preferably organic.

1. In a medium sized saucepan, put the oil and onion, cook on medium/low heat, stirring occasionally until the onion is soft, about 5 minutes. Take care not to let the onions catch and burn.
2. Add the stock, beans and zucchini. Turn the heat up to warm through.
3. Then add the leaves, so they just wilt.
4. Pour into a serving bowl and top with the parsley and caper oil, and grated cheese.

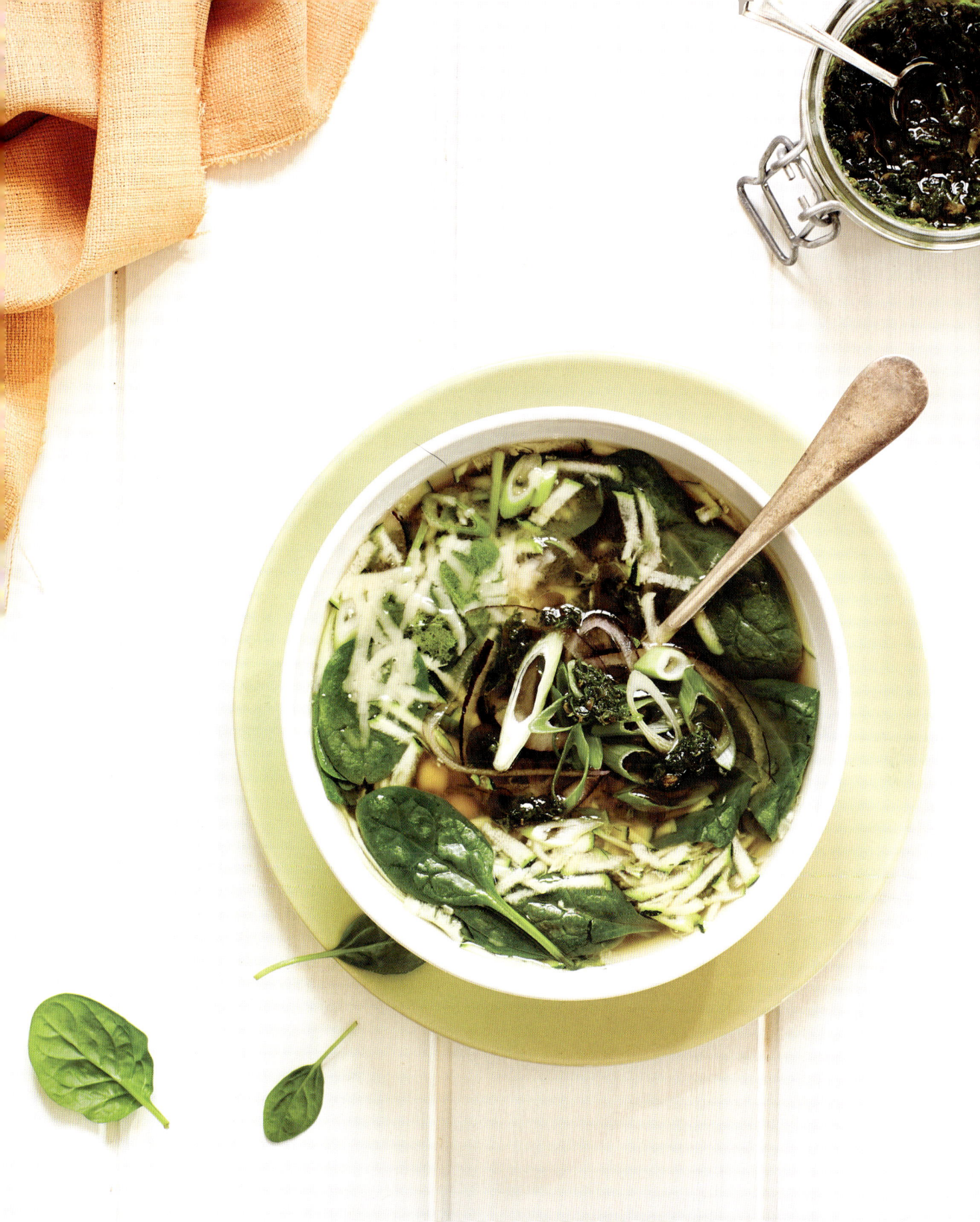

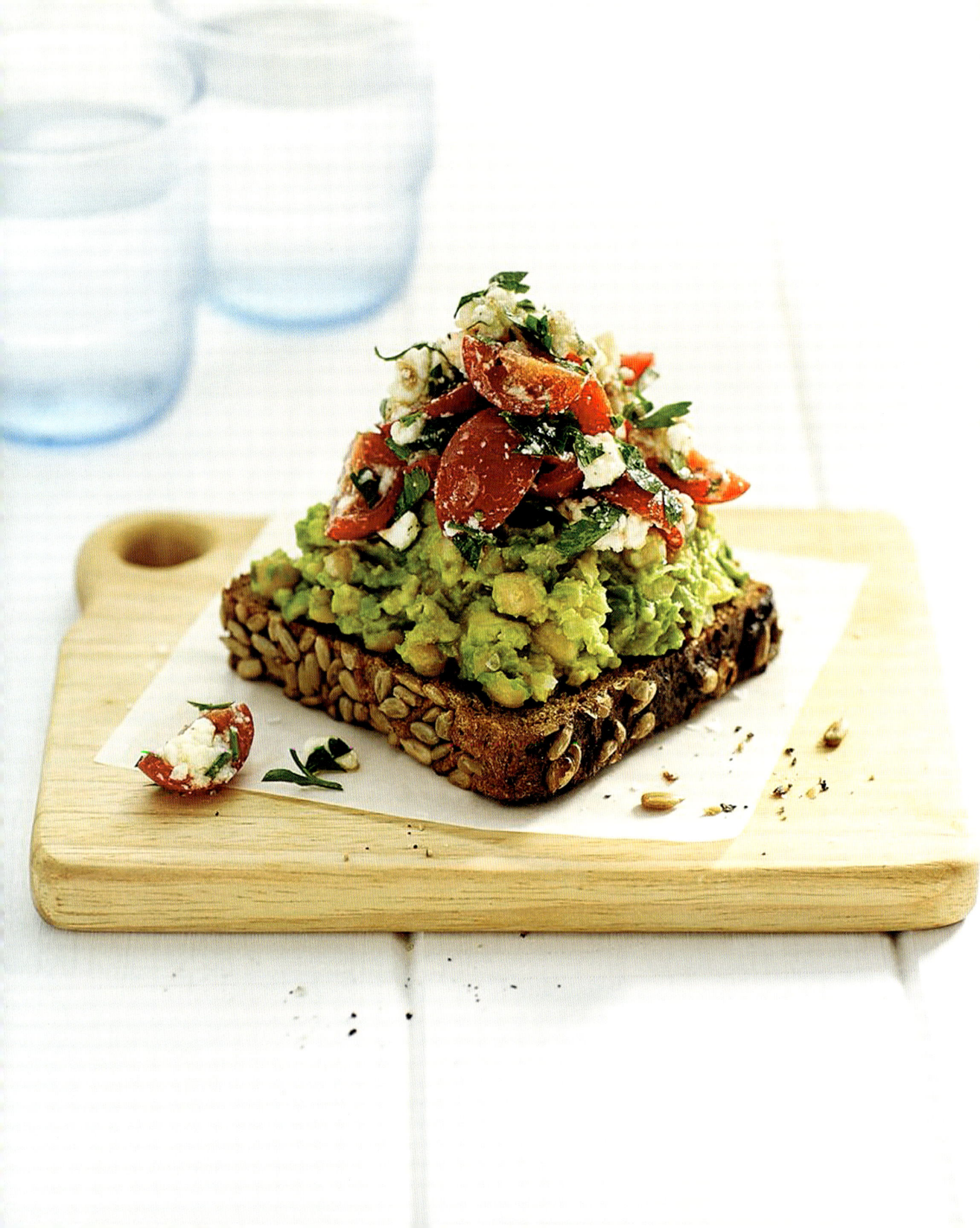

Smashed Avocado with Chickpeas, Feta and Lime (V)

Serves 1

Chickpeas provide both phytoestrogen benefits and are great fiber. They help to balance female hormones and blood sugar levels, as well as provide great food for your beneficial gut bacteria. The avocado and olive oil provide 'good' fats for female hormone balance.

INGREDIENTS
- ½ large avocado flesh
- 50 g (2 oz) cooked chickpeas (garbanzo) beans
- 1 tablespoon lime or lemon juice
- Salt and freshly ground pepper
- 20 g (1 oz) organic feta, crumbled
- 4–5 cherry tomatoes, washed and cut into quarters
- 1 tablespoon parsley, chopped
- 1 tablespoon extra virgin olive oil
- 1 slice of multi-grain sourdough or gluten-free buckwheat toast

1. In a bowl, roughly mash the avocado with the lime juice and chickpeas.
2. Add salt and pepper to taste. Then pile onto the toast or into a breakfast bowl, if you prefer not to have toast.
3. Toss the crumbled feta, olive oil, tomatoes and parsley together, season with salt and pepper. Spoon over the top of your smashed avocado.

Nourishing Broth with Ginger and Wild Mushrooms

Serves 1

This super quick recipe contains ginger, which is beneficial for its anti-inflammatory effects including on the gut itself. Spinach is high in magnesium, vitamin C and vitamin B6, all of which help alleviate some of the symptoms of PMS and menopause.

INGREDIENTS

300 ml (½ pint) homemade Chicken or Beef or Vegetable Broth (recipes pages 26–27)
100 g (3½ oz) wild mushrooms, roughly chopped
1 small knob ginger, enough to yield 1 heaped teaspoon finely grated
1 large handful baby spinach leaves, chopped kale or chopped greens, washed
1 spring onion (scallion), washed, white and green finely chopped
75 g (3 oz) firm tofu
tamari soy sauce

1. Pour the broth into a saucepan and bring to the boil, then turn down to simmer.
2. Add the mushrooms, ginger, spinach, spring onion. Stir through to warm until the spinach has wilted, about 30 seconds.
3. Pour into a serving bowl and crumble in the tofu.
4. Splash over a little tamari sauce to taste. If using bought stock, this may have salt already added.

Carrot, Leek and Borlotti Bean Soup with Parsley Oil

Serves 4

Carrots and parsley contain phytonutrients, which are used as antioxidants in the body, helping to prevent cell damage. They also contain beta-carotene, the precursor to vitamin A, which is great for ovarian health. Leeks are high in inulin, a prebiotic food for beneficial gut bacteria, which helps with better nutrient absorption and to reduce inflammation. It also supports serotonin production, the 'happy hormone'.

INGREDIENTS

Soup
- 1 tablespoon extra virgin olive oil
- 1 leek, white part only, rinsed well and finely chopped
- ½ teaspoon turmeric powder
- 1 garlic clove, peeled and crushed
- 4 carrots,
- 125 g (4½ oz) dried Borlotti beans, soaked overnight or 250 g (9 oz) of canned beans
- 1 L (32 fl oz) home made chicken broth or almond milk or vegetable stock
- Salt and freshly ground pepper

Optional: If you wish, you can use cauliflower instead of carrot.

Parsley Oil
- 4 handfuls of continental parsley leaves, washed and dried
- 2 tablespoons capers
- 125 ml (4 fl oz) extra virgin olive oil
- Pinch of salt

1. Put 1 tablespoon of olive oil and the leek into a large saucepan, on low heat. Gradually cook and soften. Put a lid on the saucepan, so the leeks sweat for about 5 minutes.
2. Add the turmeric powder and garlic and mix in. Then add the carrot and Borlotti beans and mix these. Add your stock or almond milk, so it comes to well above the mixture, and turn the heat to high. Bring to boil, then turn the heat down and simmer until the carrots and Borlotti beans are soft, about 30–40 minutes.
3. If you have some almond pulp from making almond milk, then add a couple of heaped tablespoons to your soup.
4. Once cooked, blend the soup with a stick blender in the saucepan or in a food processor. The soup may splash, as it is very hot. So take care.
5. Add salt and freshly ground pepper to taste.

To make the parsley oil:
1. When the soup is almost cooked, put the extra virgin olive oil, capers, salt and parsley into a food processor or blender. Blend until the parsley is mashed up. This could take up to 5 minutes. Stop half way and scrape down the sides with a spatula.
2. Pour the soup into bowls and add a couple of teaspoons of parsley oil to the top.

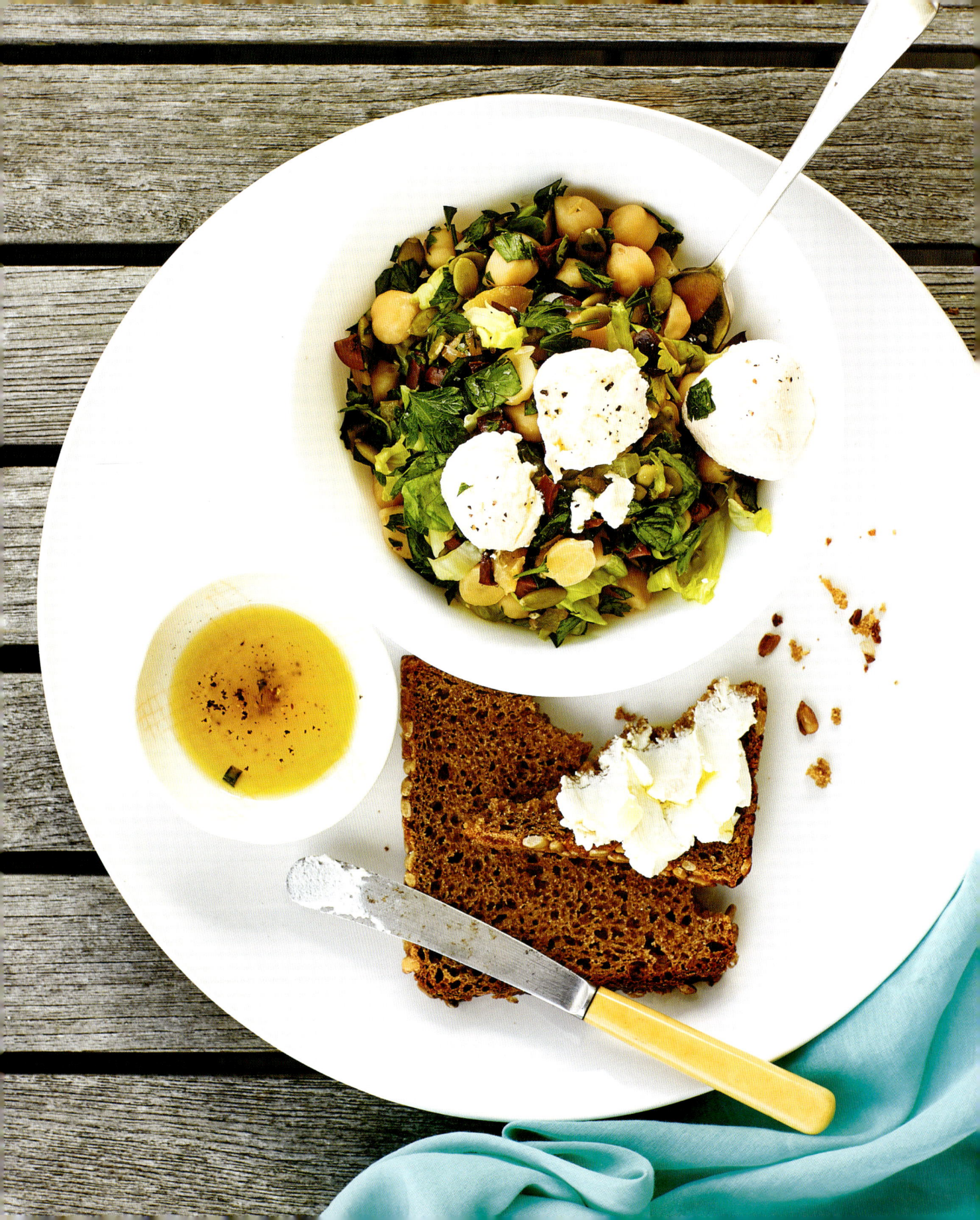

Preserved Lemon and Olive Salad with Labne (V)

Serves 2

The chickpeas in this dish provide great fiber for your beneficial gut bacteria, and that fiber makes you feel full for longer. It also helps with blood sugar regulation, in preventing constipation and clearing excess unwanted oestrogen. The parsley supports liver function, helping your liver to metabolize any unwanted toxins and female hormones. Both parsley and labne are good sources of calcium. The lovely flavors from the preserved lemon, olives and herbs help with digestion and regulating bowel movements.

INGREDIENTS

- 60 g (2 ½ oz) cooked chickpeas (cook your own or canned)
- 1 tablespoon preserved lemon flesh, finely diced. Salt removed
- 20 g (1 oz) pitted quality olives, roughly chopped
- 1 heaped tablespoon fresh thyme leaves
- 15 g (½ oz) pepita or pumpkin seeds
- 1 cos lettuce heart, washed and finely shredded
- 1 handful parsley leaves, washed and chopped
- 1 tablespoon extra virgin olive oil
- ½ lemon, juiced
- Pinch freshly ground pepper
- 6 homemade labne balls

1. Put all the salad ingredients into a bowl and toss.
2. Top with homemade Labne balls (recipe page 33) or use the balls to spread onto Sesame and Sunflower Crisp Breads (recipe page 181) and eat with the salad.

Mushroom and Buckwheat Noodle Salad (V)

Serves 2

This great tasting and digestion-stimulating salad provides:
- anti-inflammatory ginger
- iodine rich seaweed for thyroid health
- tofu, seaweed, seeds and buckwheat for phyto-oestrogen benefits
- bok choy and spinach for liver support
- Asian mushrooms for immune enhancing properties

It's an all round winner for female hormone balance and health.

INGREDIENTS

65 g (2½ oz) 100 per cent buckwheat noodles
1 tablespoon extra virgin olive oil
2 spring onions (scallions), washed and finely sliced diagonally
1 x 3 cm (1½ inch) knob of fresh ginger (no need to peel) washed and finely grated
½ long red chili, de-seeded and finely chopped
1 handful shiitake mushrooms, sliced
1 handful enoki mushrooms
2 handfuls spinach or bok choy, washed
1 heaped tablespoon dried arame seaweed, reconstituted with hot water, as per packet instructions
2 teaspoons pickled ginger, finely sliced (recipe page 35)
100 g (3½ oz) firm organic tofu, crumbled
2 teaspoons sesame seeds
1 tablespoon pepita seeds
2 teaspoons sesame oil
2 teaspoons umeboshi plum vinegar or 1 umeboshi plum, finely chopped

1. Place the noodles in a large saucepan of salted boiling water and cook until just done, about 6 minutes. Then drain and put into a bowl of cold water.
2. In a frying pan, skillet or wok, on medium heat, in the oil, cook the spring onions, fresh ginger and chili until the onion has turned bright green, about 1 minute.
3. Add the mushrooms and green leaves, tossing until just wilting, about 30 seconds. Put into a bowl to cool.
4. Drain the noodles and seaweed and add to the bowl of mushrooms.
5. Add the pickled ginger, tofu, sesame seeds, pepitas, sesame oil and umeboshi vinegar/plum. Then, using your hands, gently mix all the ingredients together and divide into 2 serving bowls.

Note: Buckwheat is a gluten-free grain. If you're not coeliac then you can use a blend of buckwheat and wheat noodles, if you wish.

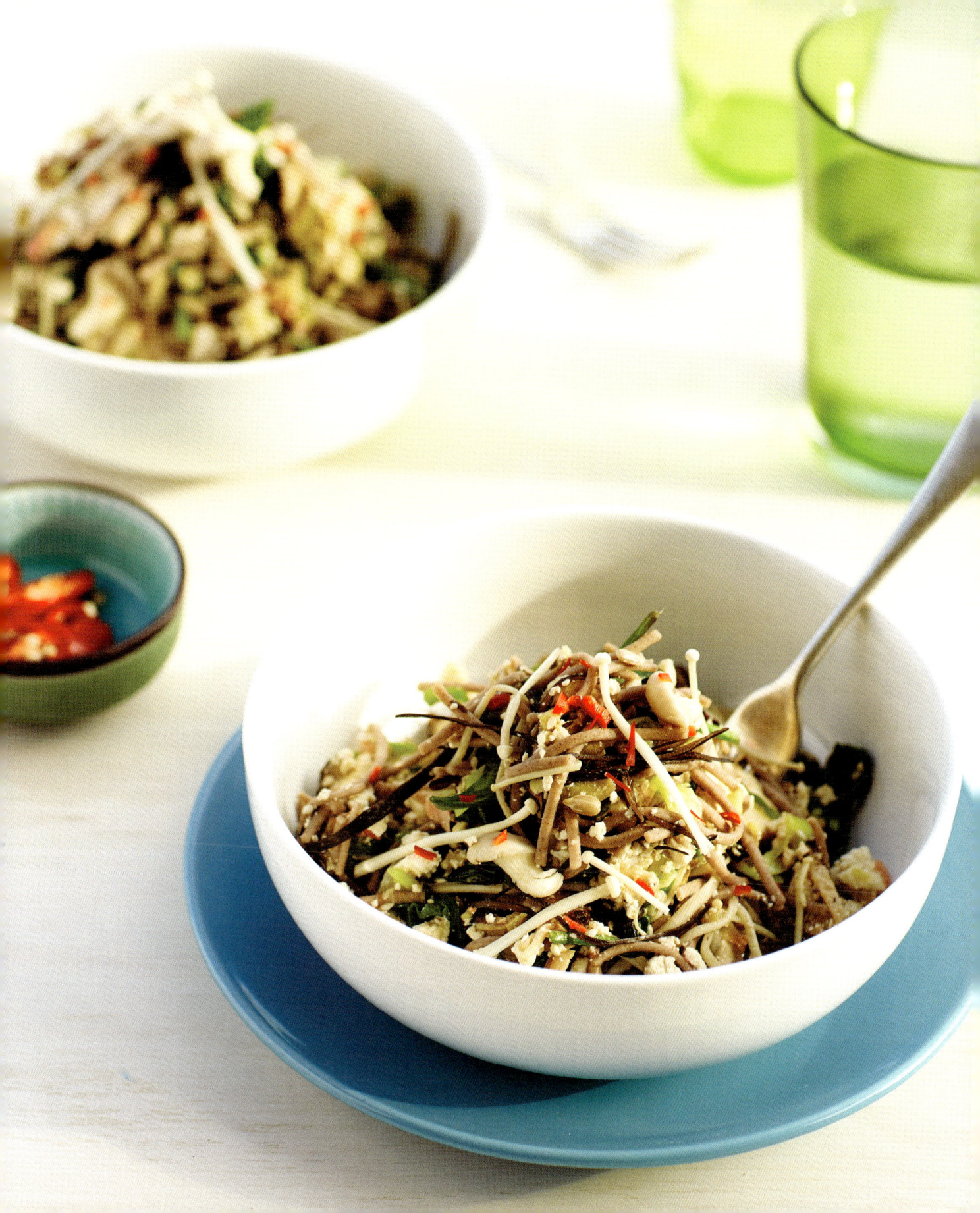

Apple and Fennel Slaw (V)

Serves 4

Research, along with traditional ayurvedic medicine, has shown that fennel seeds have some benefit in helping reduce menstrual cramps. The cabbage helps support oestrogen clearance from the liver further relieving symptoms of PMS. The phytoestrogen in cabbage helps reduce many of the menopausal symptoms. Cabbage also contains boron, vitamin C and calcium which help support bone health.

INGREDIENTS

- 2 tablespoons lemon juice
- 2 tablespoons extra virgin olive oil
- 1 large apple
- 2 large carrots
- 200 g (7 oz) red cabbage
- 1 teaspoon fennel seeds
- 2 handfuls of parsley, chopped
- Salt and pepper

1. Mix the lemon juice and olive oil in a salad bowl.
2. Wash the apple. Leaving the skin on, coarsely grate it into the oil and lemon juice. Toss to coat the apple.
3. Wash and peel the carrots, if they aren't organic. Then coarsely grate into the bowl.
4. Wash the cabbage and finely shred, using a sharp knife or mandolin.
5. Add the cabbage to the bowl, along with the fennel seeds and parsley.
6. Mix all the ingredients together well, avoiding any clumps of one type of vegetable.
7. Serve this with Chicken and Lentil Burgers (recipe page 81) and Tzatziki (recipe page 178).

·Chicken and Lentil Burgers· *Makes 5 burgers*

These burgers contain phytoestrogens in both the lentils and tofu, which help to modulate the effects of oestrogen. The lentils also provide excellent fiber to nourish your beneficial bacteria in the gut, assisting it to function more effectively in absorbing nutrients. They support serotonin production, a 'good mood' neurotransmitter.

The chicken provides a good source of vitamin B6, which helps with the production of neurotransmitters. These play a key role in mood, pain, depression and anxiety management. B6 may also help with fluid retention around the time of menstruation.

INGREDIENTS

- 300 g (10 oz) chicken mince or salmon fillet mince, if you prefer
- 120 g (4 oz) firm tofu, finely crumbled
- 100 g (3 oz) cooked orange lentils (cook your own or canned)
- 1 teaspoon turmeric powder
- 1 heaped teaspoon garam masala
- Big pinch cayenne pepper
- 2 tablespoons coconut oil, warmed and runny
- ¼ teaspoon salt
- 3 spring onions, finely chopped
- 1 ripe avocado, thinly sliced

1. In a bowl, using your hands, mix together the mince, tofu, lentils, spices, salt, onions and 1 tablespoon of oil. Smash up the lentils as you mix. Then squash and press the mixture together so it forms one sticky mass.
2. Roll into 5 balls and flatten each ball into a burger shape.
3. Heat a frying pan/skillet on medium, add 1 tablespoon of coconut oil and fry the burgers for 3–4 minutes on each side until the mince in the center has cooked.
4. Eat with the Apple and Fennel Slaw (recipe page 80), Tzatziki (recipe page 178) and topped with fresh avocado slices. You can pile all this into a multigrain bun or pita pocket.

Note: If you wish to cook these later, you can chill the burgers and use the next day.

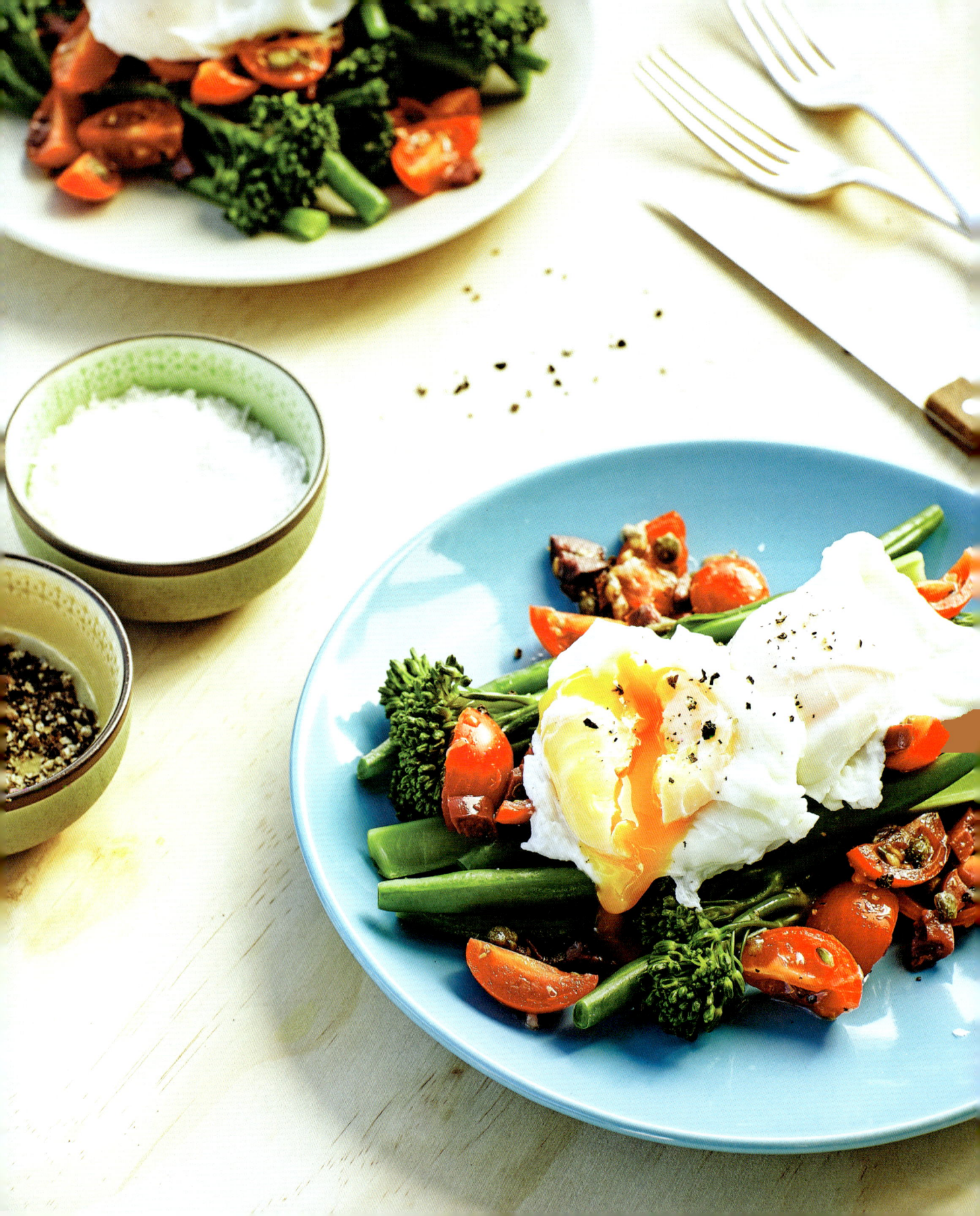

Puttanesca Green Beans and Broccolini with Poached Eggs (V)

Serves 2

The flavors in this nourishing quick lunch stimulate digestion and offer their own blend of beneficial phytonutrients. The broccolini provides liver support to help process some of the symptoms of menopause (see page 9).

INGREDIENTS

- 150 g (5 oz) broccolini or tenderstem broccoli
- 170 g (6 oz) french green beans or round beans with woody stem trimmed
- 1 tablespoon capers
- 1 preserved/pickled anchovy fillet
- 1 small garlic clove, peeled and crushed
- 5 black Kalamatta olives, pitted
- 1 handful cherry tomatoes, halved
- 1 tablespoon extra virgin olive oil
- ½ lemon, juiced
- Pinch salt and freshly ground pepper
- 4 organic free-range eggs (2 eggs per person)

1. Steam the broccolini and green beans for 4 minutes until just cooked and retaining a little bit of crunch. Put into a mixing bowl.
2. Roughly chop the capers, olives and anchovy. Add to the mixing bowl and toss with the garlic, tomatoes, lemon, oil and pepper.
3. Divide the bean mixture between two serving plates.
4. Bring the water you used to steam the vegetables to just simmering and poach the eggs for 2–3 minutes or until the egg white is cooked, but the yolk is still soft.
5. Take out of the water and place on top of the vegetables. Sprinkle salt and pepper on the eggs, and enjoy.

Red Onion Tart with Herb Salad (V)

Tart serves 6–8 / Salad serves 4

Onions are part of the Allium family of vegetables, known for their beneficial high polyphenol phytonutrient (antioxidant plant nutrient) content. Their sulfur compounds are great for your liver and gut. They act as a prebiotic, a specialized plant fiber which nourishes the 'good' bacteria in your gut.

The high flavonoid (plant pigment) antioxidant content, in particular, quercetin, acts as an anti-inflammatory in your body. This is what gives the onions their red color.

Peel as little of the skin off the red onions as the highest concentration of their beneficial flavonoid nutrients are found in the outer layers.

INGREDIENTS

Pastry
200 g (7 oz) frozen or cold buckwheat flour* or whole wheat flour
125 g (4½ oz) cold organic butter, chopped
Pinch of salt
3 tablespoons cold water

Filling
4 large red onions, peeled and each cut into 8 wedges
½ tablespoon extra virgin olive oil
Salt and freshly ground pepper
2 large organic free range eggs, beaten
250 g (9 oz) natural unsweetened yogurt (goat, sheep, organic cow's or buffalo)
1 tablespoon fresh thyme leaves, washed
1 garlic clove, peeled and crushed
60 g (2½ oz) pitted black Kalamata olives, roughly chopped
2 tablespoons feta, crumbled

Salad
1 bunch continental/flat leaf parsley, washed and leaves roughly chopped
1 bunch mint, washed and leaves roughly chopped
80 g (3 oz) cooked lentils
300 g (10½ oz) cherry tomatoes, washed and cut into quarters

Dressing
1 tablespoon apple cider vinegar
2 tablespoons extra virgin olive oil
Pinch salt and freshly ground pepper

1. Set your oven to 180°C (350°F) fan forced or 200°C (390°F) regular.
2. In a bowl, toss the onions with olive oil and a pinch of salt and pepper.
3. Put the onions onto a baking tray lined with baking/parchment paper, then into the oven for about 20–30 minutes or until just soft.

Continued on page 87

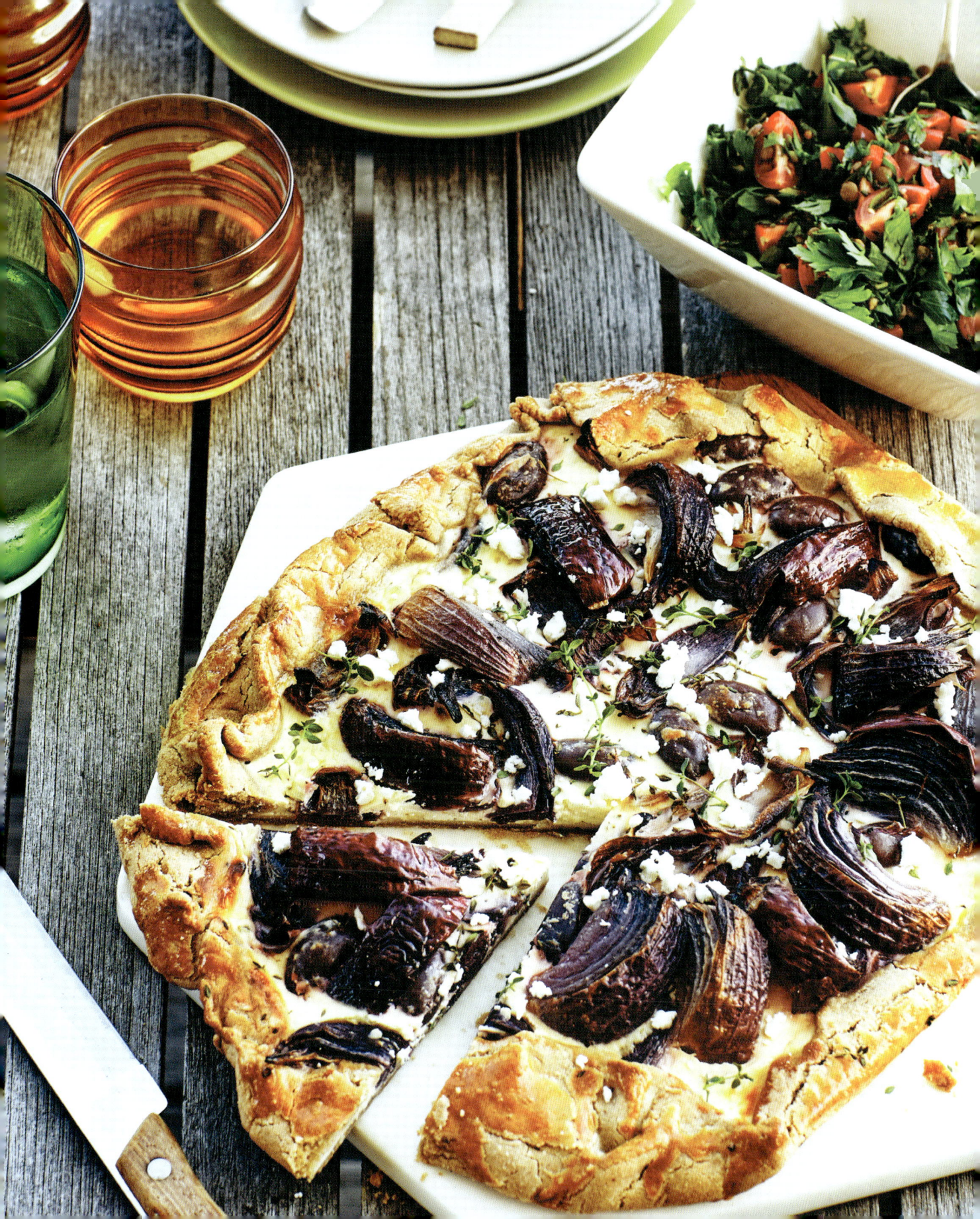

To make the pastry:
1. Put the cold flour, salt and butter into a food processor. Blend until the mixture is like breadcrumbs, about 30 seconds.
2. With the motor running, add the cold water and process until the pastry comes together into a ball, about 1 minute.
3. Remove and place onto a floured surface. Roll out into a rough circle about 30 cm (12 inch) in diameter. This can be as misshapen as you like, since this is a free-form pie. Any shape is good!
4. Carefully move onto another baking tray lined with baking/parchment paper. If any of the pastry flops over the side, that's okay as you will fold it in once the filling is made.

To make the filling:
1. In a bowl combine the eggs and yogurt. Roughly mix together. Add the thyme, garlic and olives and mix.
2. Pour this mixture into the center of the pastry, place the onions on top, with some of them poking up, 'soldiers-on-parade-style'. Spread the filling ingredients leaving about 2.5 cm (1 inch) gap around the edges.
3. Scatter the feta over the filling.
4. Fold over the edges of the tart 'free-form' style.
5. Put the tart into the oven to bake for 35 minutes.
6. Make up the salad dressing in a salad bowl. Toss in the salad ingredients and mix together.
7. Once the tart is cooked, the pastry will be quite soft whilst it is very hot. Leave it for 10 minutes before cutting it up. Serve with the salad.

Note: Buckwheat flour is gluten-free.

Watercress, Broccolini and Walnut Salad (V)

Serves 2

Watercress and broccolini are great sources of vitamin C which helps boost your energy, as well as bone health. They are also rich in vitamin K and calcium. Watercress is high in beta-carotene (which is converted to vitamin A in your body), which gives mucus membrane support, especially during menopause. Your liver loves the indole-3-carbinols derived from the breakdown of the sulfur-containing compounds in broccolini. This helps to relieve symptoms of PMS and menopause.

INGREDIENTS

- 1 bunch broccolini, washed and trimmed
- A large handful of watercress, washed and roughly chopped
- 3 stalks of celery, washed and thinly sliced
- 2–3 tablespoons Labne (recipe page 33), soft goat cheese or 4 tablespoons organic ricotta
- 2 tablespoons roughly chopped walnuts
- 1 tablespoon sunflower seeds
- Salt and freshly ground pepper to taste
- ½ lemon, juiced

1. Blanch or steam the broccolini until just tender, about 3–4 minutes. Take the broccolini out of the water/steamer and immediately plunge into cold water to stop the cooking. Drain the broccolini and carefully shake out any excess water that has clung to the flower head.
2. Toss all the ingredients together in a bowl, massaging the goat cheese into the vegetables with your hands.

DIY Rice Paper Rolls with Avocado and Mint

Makes about 12. Serves 4

Cabbage belongs to the brassica family and these vegetables are powerful supporters in detoxification in your liver. The avocado provides good fats to 'feed' your ovaries. The coriander and mint aid digestion and liver functions, as well as taste great! There's plenty of fiber found in the lentils, which help to keep both the liver and gut happy, leading to happy balanced hormones.

INGREDIENTS

100 g (3½ oz) finely sliced wombok (Chinese cabbage)
1 large ripe avocado, stone and skin removed, finely sliced
½ long red chili, split in half lengthways, seeds scraped out, finely chopped
1 small handful of fresh mint, washed and finely chopped
1 small handful of coriander (cilantro) leaves, washed and finely chopped
1 handful sprouted green lentils
2 tablespoons finely chopped pickled ginger (recipe page 35)
1 packet rice papers – 19 cm x 19 cm (7.5 inch x 7.5 inch) or similar round size

Dressing
3 tablespoons rice vinegar
3 tablespoons tamari soy sauce

Additional options
Cooked peeled prawns
Firm organic tofu
Homemade nut butter or
Shredded chicken

1. This is fun when you get together with some girlfriends. Put everything on a table and make up your rolls as you go.
2. Alternatively, mix the wombok, avocado, chili, mint, coriander, lentils and ginger in a bowl.
3. Place a clean tea towel onto the kitchen bench, with the bowl of salad to one side, your protein to the other and a tray in front of you.
4. In a large bowl with hot water, submerge a piece of rice paper for about 12 seconds or until it softens.
5. Take it out of the water and lay it flat on the tea towel.
6. Put a couple of tablespoons of salad ingredients into the first ⅓ of the paper. Top this with your choice of protein — prawn, shredded chicken, slice of tofu or a dollop of nut butter.
7. Bring in both sides of the paper to fold partly over the ingredients.
8. Then roll up your rice paper parcel as tightly as you can without the paper splitting. Pop onto your tray. Repeat until all the filling and protein has gone.
9. Make the dressing in a bowl for dipping.
10. If you wish, these rolls will keep wrapped in the fridge for the next day.

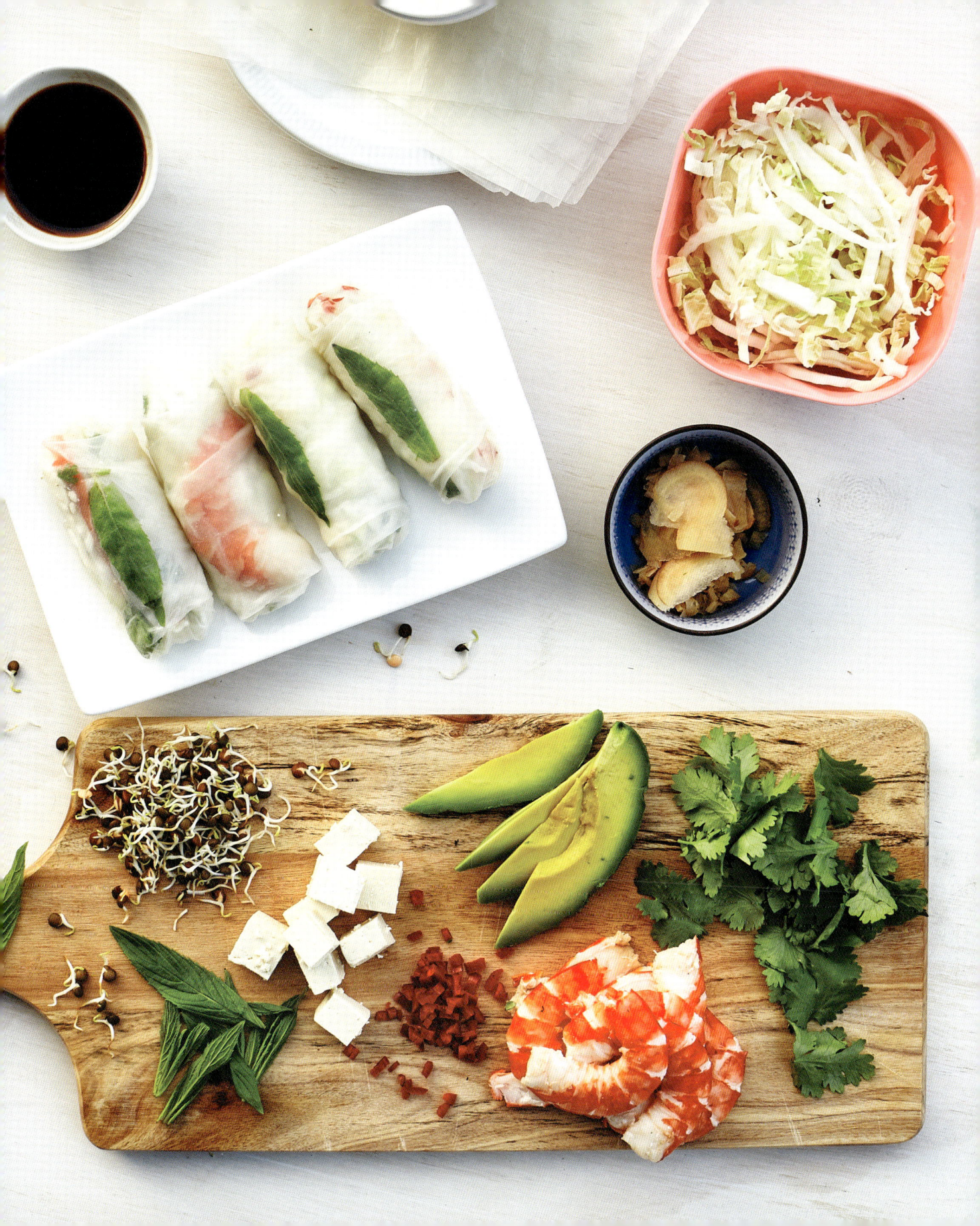

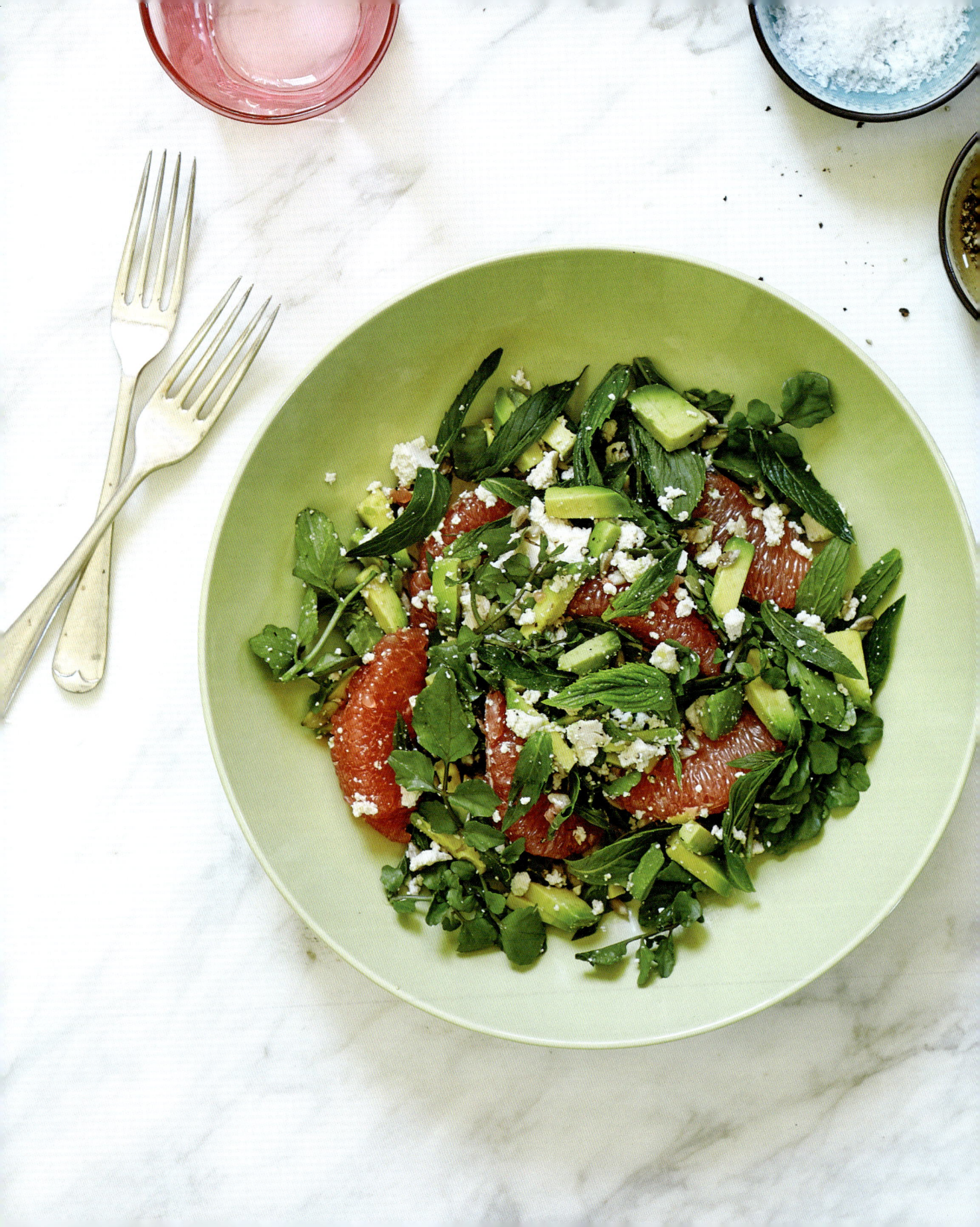

Ruby Grapefruit and Mint Salad (V)

Serves 1

Whist the tofu and seeds provide beneficial phytoestrogens, the red grapefruit is a good source of the phytonutrients, lycopene and limonoids. These help promote a detoxifying enzyme in the liver that helps make toxic compounds, such as xenoestrogens and 'used' hormones, more water soluble and, therefore, more easily excreted.

INGREDIENTS

- A big handful of fresh watercress leaves, washed
- 1 handful fresh mint leaves, washed
- 1 small avocado or half a large, deseeded and peeled
- 1 ruby grapefruit, peeled, segmented and roughly chopped, pips removed
- 60 g (2½ oz) firm organic tofu, crumbled
- 1 tablespoon pepita or pumpkin seeds
- 1 tablespoon sunflower seeds
- 1 tablespoon extra virgin olive oil
- 1 tablespoon apple cider vinegar
- Big pinch salt and freshly ground pepper

1. Toss everything together in a bowl and enjoy.

Big Mug of Goodness (V)

Serves 1

This recipe is super fast to make and full of goodness. It has a great fermented benefit in the miso paste, as well as quality phytoestrogens in the miso and tofu. The folic acid in the spinach helps your body repair and produce new cells and in the synthesis of serotonin, one of the happy hormones.

INGREDIENTS

- 2–3 heaped teaspoons organic miso paste (check the recommended quantity on the packet)
- 500 ml (16 fl oz) boiling water
- 1 handful baby spinach, washed
- 80 g (3 oz) firm organic tofu, crumbled
- 2 heaped tablespoons shiitake or other Asian-style mushrooms, finely sliced
- 1 spring onion (scallion), washed and finely chopped
- ½ cm (¼ inch) knob of fresh ginger
- pinch fresh long green chili, de-seeded and finely chopped or pinch dried chili flakes
- 1 teaspoon sesame seeds

1. Get all your ingredients together first.
2. Spoon the miso paste into your big mug. Stir in the boiling water and mix using a fork, until fully dissolved.
3. Add the spinach and stir until it wilts. Add the tofu, onions and mushrooms. Grate in the fresh ginger and add the chili. The amount is up to you.
4. Sprinkle over the sesame seeds and enjoy.

Note: Choose bright, vibrant-looking green spinach leaves, as research shows this indicates greater levels of vitamin C which helps protect the beneficial phytonutrients in the leaves from oxidation damage. Interestingly, baby spinach leaves stored in sealed bags exposed to store lighting, can keep their vitamin C stable for up to 9 days, if also kept at a low temperature of 4°C (39°F).

Ginger and Edamame Turmeric Fried Rice

Serves 1

This is a comfort food dish. Not only is it easy to digest, it is very satisfying.

The phytoestrogens and fiber in this dish help modulate and excrete oestrogen. The turmeric, coriander, garlic, ginger and cabbage assist the liver's detoxification processes, for all round body and mind health, not just female hormone balance.

INGREDIENTS

- 1 tablespoon extra virgin olive oil
- 2 tablespoons sesame seeds
- 1 large spring onion (scallion), washed and finely chopped
- 100 g (3½ oz) wombok (Chinese cabbage), thinly sliced
- 1 stick celery, washed and finely sliced
- 100 g (3½ oz) cooked brown rice
- 45 g (2 oz) fresh or frozen soya beans (weight once removed from their pods)
- 3 cm (2 inch) knob of fresh unpeeled turmeric, washed and grated or 1 level teaspoon turmeric powder
- 1 heaped tablespoon fresh unpeeled ginger, coarsely grated
- 1 small clove of garlic, peeled and crushed
- 1 handful fresh coriander (cilantro) leaves, washed and roughly chopped
- 1 tablespoon brown rice vinegar
- Soy or tamari sauce
- Cooked meat or fish or 2 eggs

1. If your rice is not already cooked, then cook 50 g (2 oz) of uncooked rice first. This will take approximately 40 minutes. Follow the instructions on the packet.
2. Have it ready before you start to put the rice mixture together.
3. In a wok/frying pan/skillet toss the olive oil, sesame seeds, soy beans, onion, wombok and celery on high heat for 2 minutes, toasting the seeds slightly.
4. Then add the rice, turmeric, ginger, garlic and coriander to the pan. Toss around to mix and warm all ingredients. Sprinkle over the rice vinegar and put into a serving bowl.
5. Add a dash of soy or tamari sauce to add saltiness to the dish.
6. If you wish, you can shred some meat or fish through the dish or place 2 cooked eggs on top after serving.

Wakame Seaweed Salad with Crunchy Tofu (V) — Serves 1

Seaweed, tofu and brown rice contain phytoestrogens, which help reduce symptoms of menopause and PMS. Seaweed also contains good levels of iodine, which helps support the thyroid function involved in metabolism and energy production. Ginger acts as an anti-inflammatory, beneficial in reducing menstrual cramps and menstrual bleeding. Tofu and the seeds contain calcium. Research has found that women suffering from PMS can have low levels of calcium. Calcium supports bone mineral formation throughout a woman's life.

INGREDIENTS

Salad
100 g (3½ oz) cooked brown rice
13 g (½ oz) dried organic Wakame
80 g (3 oz) cucumber, thinly sliced
12 g (½ oz) pickled ginger, finely shredded (recipe page 35)
1 celery stalk, washed and finely sliced
20 g (1 oz) hemp or sesame seeds

Tofu
30 g (1 oz) brown rice flour
120 g (4½ oz) firm organic tofu, cut into 8 cubes
1 teaspoon extra virgin olive oil

Dressing
1 teaspoon organic miso paste
1 tablespoon rice vinegar
1 tablespoon extra virgin olive oil

1. If your rice is not already cooked, then cook 50 g (2 oz) uncooked weight, first. This will take approximately 40 minutes. Follow the instructions on the packet.
2. Soak the Wakame in water for 10 minutes, then drain. This should make up 85 g (3 oz) of seaweed.
3. Mix the dressing ingredients together in a small salad bowl for one. Add the cooked rice, Wakame, cucumber, pickled ginger, celery and seeds, but don't mix them together.
4. Toss the tofu in the rice flour. Add 1 teaspoon of olive to a small frying pan/skillet and heat to medium-low. Once warm, add the tofu and crisp for 20 seconds on each side.
5. Mix the salad together and place the tofu on top.

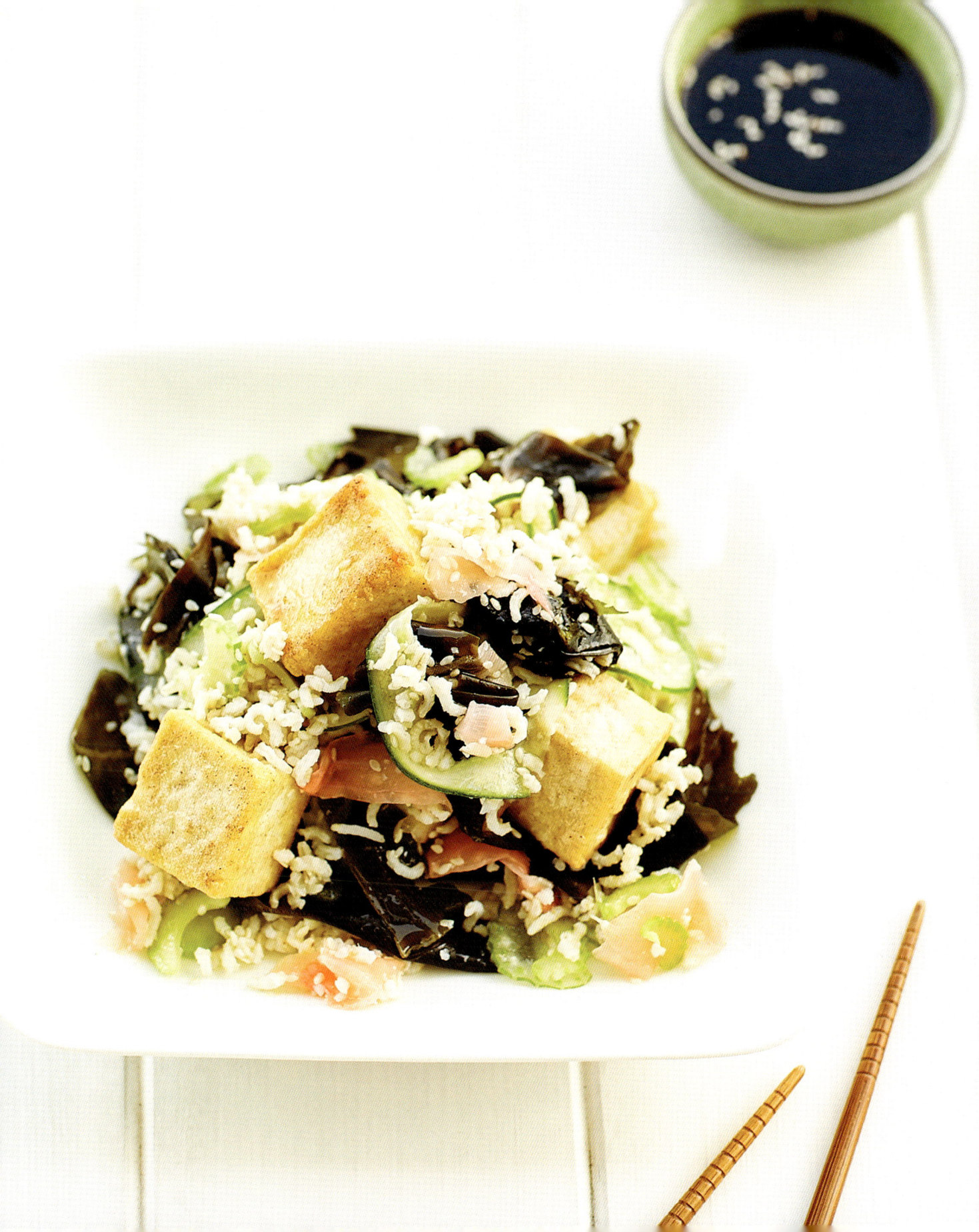

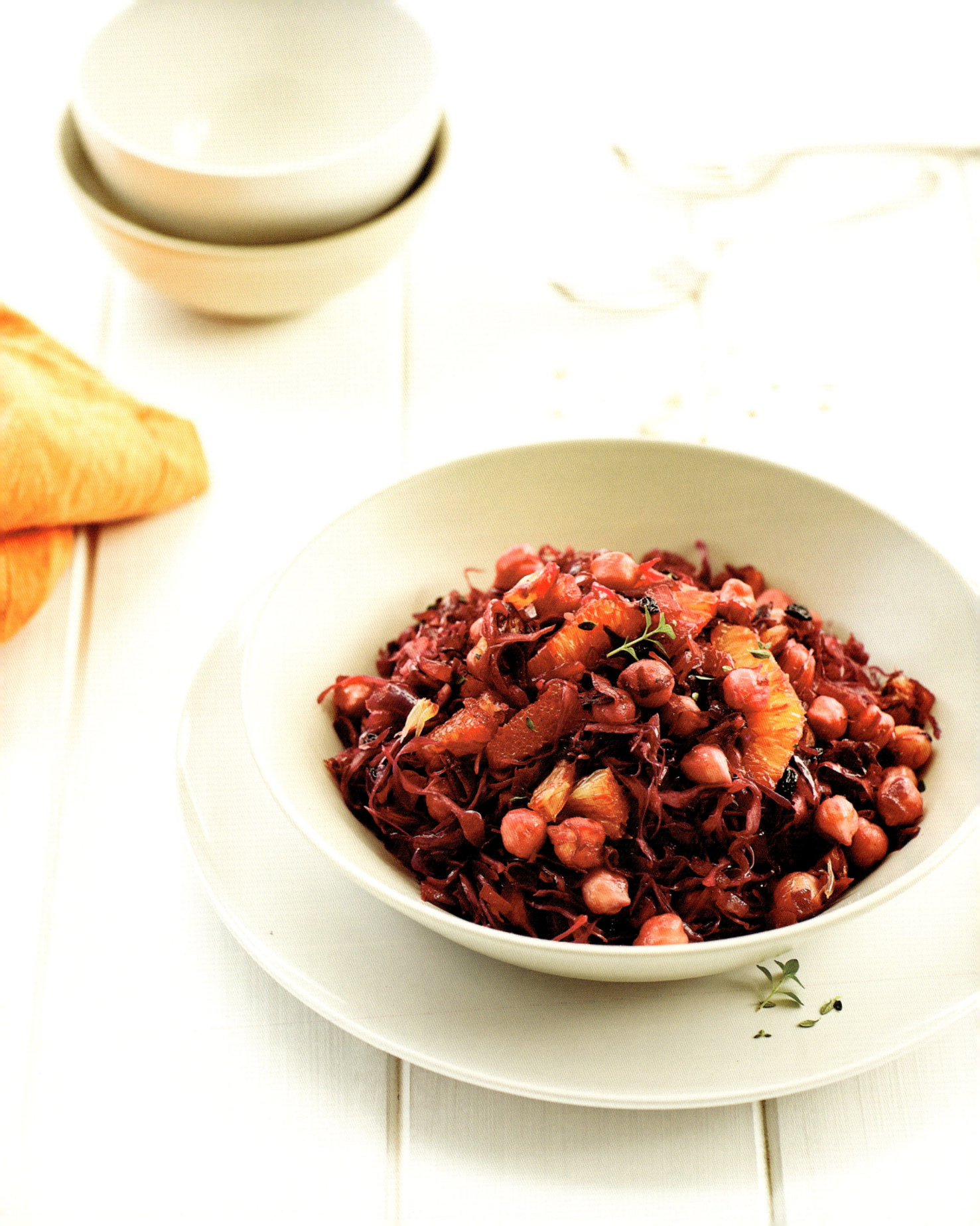

Warm Beetroot, Chickpea and Red Cabbage Salad (V)

Serves 2, with some leftovers

Cabbage, a brassica vegetable, contains potent oestrogen balancing properties. This supports the liver to 'mop up' excess oestrogen and helps relieve associated problems such as PMS, acne, weight gain as well as symptoms of menopause

INGREDIENTS

- 2 tablespoons almonds, roughly chopped
- 2 tablespoons extra virgin olive oil
- 1 red onion, finely diced
- 60 g (3 oz) beetroot, washed and coarsely grated (no need to peel)
- ¼ red cabbage, finely shredded
- 1 tablespoon dried currants
- 1 orange, peeled and segmented with any pips removed
- 100 g (3½ oz) cooked chickpeas (cook your own or canned)
- 1 tablespoon fresh or 1 teaspoon dried thyme
- 1 tablespoon apple cider vinegar
- Big pinch salt and freshly ground pepper

1. If you are cooking the chickpeas, soak them overnight in cold water and cook for approximately 30 minutes or until just soft.
2. Toast the almonds in a large frying pan on a gentle heat for a few minutes. Remove and leave to cool.
3. In the pan, on a gentle heat, in 2 tablespoons of olive oil, fry the onion until just softening, about 5 minutes.
4. Add the beetroot and cook until it softens. Add the cabbage. Toss it until it is just wilted, about 1 minute.
5. Place the beetroot and cabbage mixture into a large serving bowl. Add the remaining ingredients, currants, orange, chickpeas, thyme, apple cider vinegar and salt and pepper, to the bowl and gently combine.

Salmon and Turmeric Broth • Serves 1

This bowl of broth really feels like it is nourishing you all through your insides! The turmeric is thought, in Traditional Chinese Medicine, to decongest the liver and reduce menstrual pain. In Western medicine, it is thought to act as an anti-inflammatory which helps to reduce PMS and menopausal symptoms.

INGREDIENTS

- 500 ml (16 fl oz) chicken bone broth (recipe page 26)
- 1 stalk of lemongrass about 8 cm (3 inch) long
- 110 g (4 oz) fresh raw salmon filet, cut into small bite size pieces
- 50 g (2 oz) sliced mushrooms, preferably shiitake
- ½ teaspoon turmeric powder or 1 teaspoon fresh grated turmeric, if you have it
- 1 big spring onion (scallion), washed and finely sliced
- 1 large handful baby spinach leaves or other green leaves, well washed
- 60 g (2 oz) cooked quinoa or brown rice
- tamari or soy sauce

1. Bash the lemongrass stalk with the back of your kitchen knife to break open the fibers.
2. Heat the broth, with the lemongrass and turmeric, so it comes to the boil. Turn off the heat.
3. Throw in the rest of the ingredients and stir gently until the spinach has wilted.
4. Pour into a serving bowl and pull out the lemongrass. You can suck on it as you eat the soup to get more of its delicate flavor, if you wish.
5. Splash in a little soy or tamari sauce, if you like it a bit salty.

Enjoy the good feeling this broth gives you! You made it with love for your body.

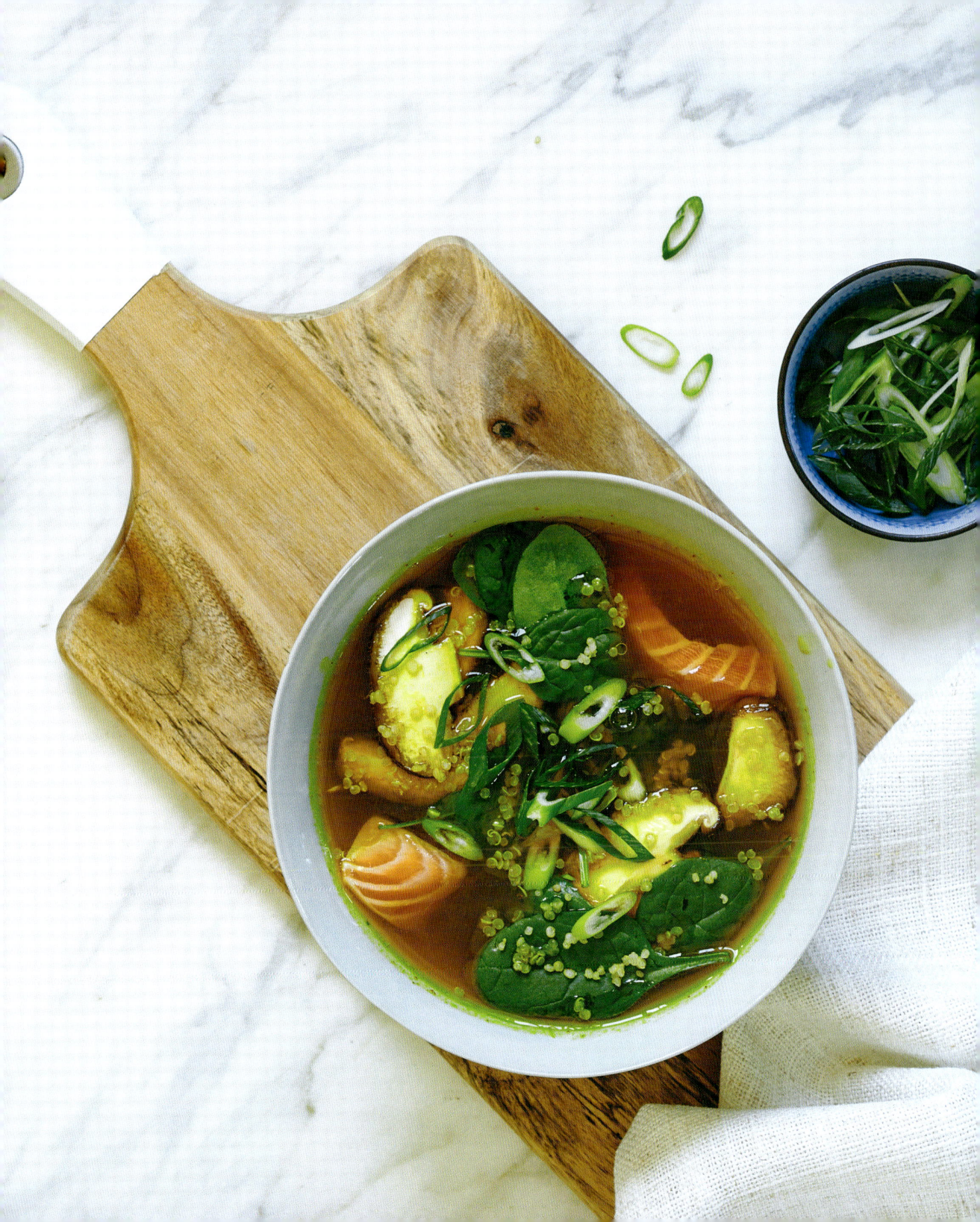

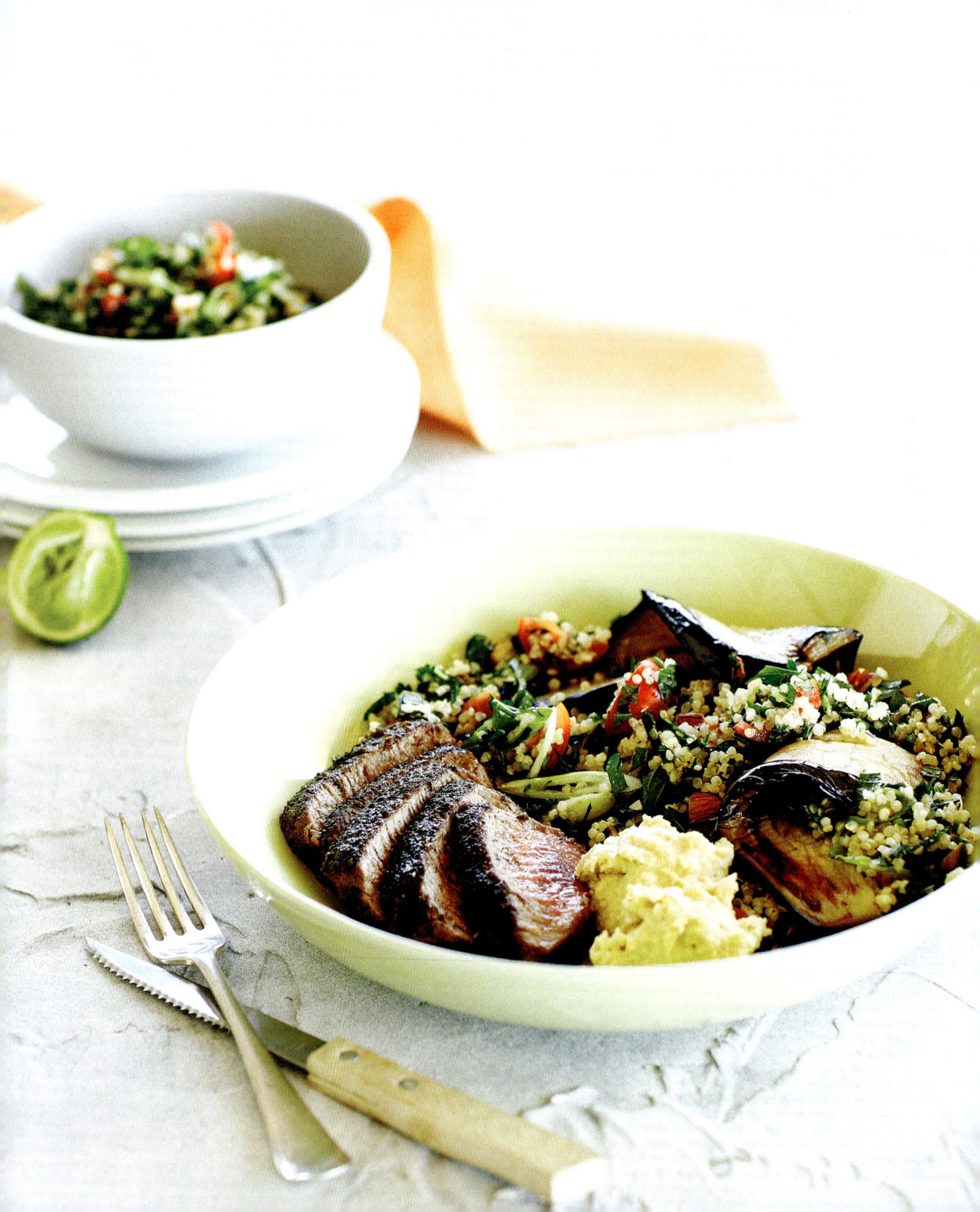

DINNER

Wok-tossed Prawns, Spinach and Brown Rice *Serves 4*

A quick and really tasty stirfry, which provides great prebiotic food from the inulin found in asparagus. This helps our gut to function better, which means more of the 'happy' hormone, serotonin, is being produced. The vegetables and fiber help our liver's detoxification work, assisting female hormone balance.

INGREDIENTS

- 400 g (14 oz) cooked brown rice or quinoa
- 1 bunch asparagus
- ½ bunch coriander (cilantro)
- 2 tablespoons coconut oil
- 3 spring onions (scallions), washed and finely chopped
- ½ fresh long red chili, de-seeded and finely chopped
- ½ red pepper (capsicum), washed, de-seeded and finely sliced
- 2 fresh or dried kaffir lime leaves
- 100 ml (3½ oz) coconut milk
- 2 big handfuls spinach or bok choy leaves, washed
- 2 cm (1 inch) cubed knob of ginger, washed and finely sliced into strips
- 1 fresh lime, quartered
- 220 g (8 oz) peeled raw prawns
- Pinch salt and freshly ground pepper
- Soy or tamari sauce

1. If starting with raw brown rice, cook 100 g (3½ oz) first to get the quantity required.
2. Gently wash the asparagus and break off the woody end of the stalk. Generally, this is about ⅓ of the asparagus spear, depending on how fresh it is.
3. Cut the asparagus spears in half and then in half lengthwise.
4. Wash the coriander well, and chop up the roots and half the lower end of the stalks. Save the leaves for later.
5. Put 1 tablespoon of coconut oil in a large fry pan or wok and turn the heat to medium.
6. If the kaffir leaves are fresh, remove the woody center vein and very finely slice. Then add the onions, chili, capsicum, asparagus, coriander roots and stalks.
7. Toss for 2 minutes. Add the brown rice, coconut milk, spinach or bok choy and ginger.
8. Gently stir this around the pan until the spinach has just wilted and the rice warmed. Turn off the heat and leave in the pan while you cook the prawns.
9. In a separate pan on high, melt the other tablespoon of coconut oil. Add the prawns and stir until cooked, about 2 minutes. Add a pinch of salt and pepper and toss through the prawns.
10. Spoon the rice and spinach mix onto serving plates. Divide the prawns amongst them and squeeze over the lime juice. Scatter the coriander leaves and splash some soy or tamari to taste.

This mouthwatering dish is great to serve for your girlfriends!

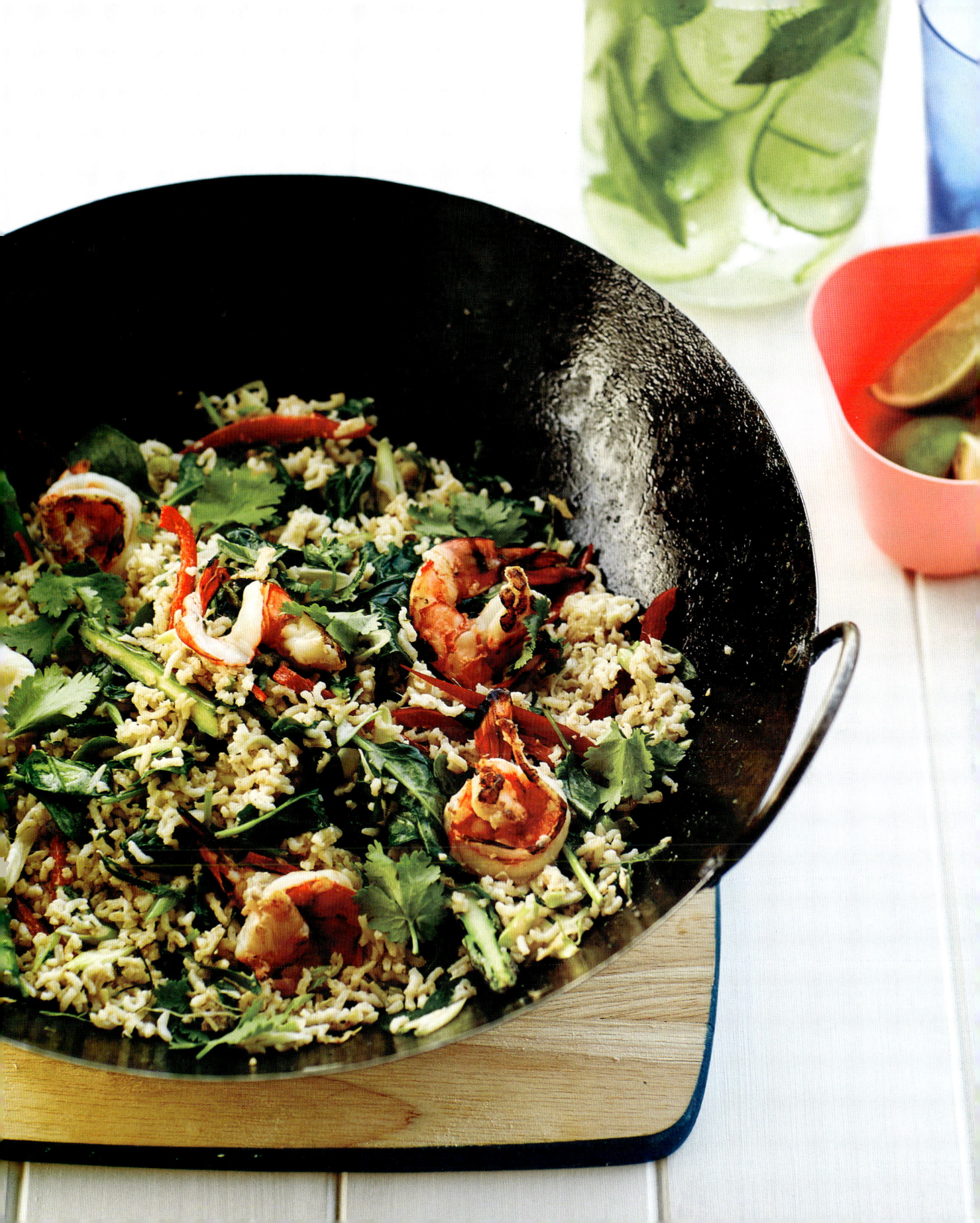

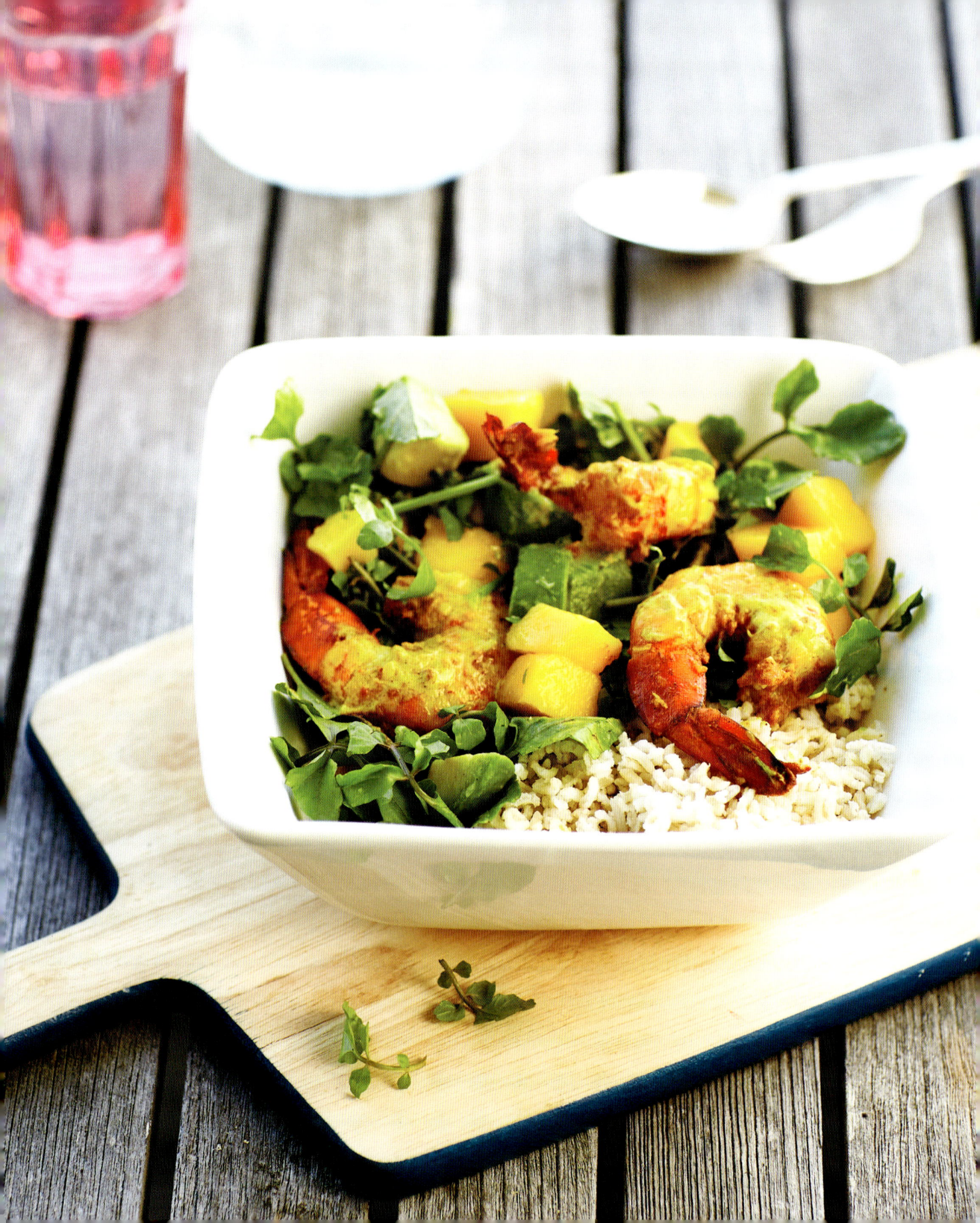

Watercress and Mango Salad with Turmeric Prawns

Serves 2

Full of phytonutrients, this dish helps with both inflammation and energy production throughout our bodies. The prawns contain the mineral selenium, which is used throughout our bodies in many processes, including liver detoxification. Reduced oestrogen following menopause may cause a reduction in selenium, accelerating the aging process, so it is an important mineral to maintain!

INGREDIENTS

- 210 g (7½ oz) cooked brown rice
- 220 g (8 oz) peeled raw prawns
- 2 tablespoons extra virgin olive oil or 1 tablespoon warmed coconut oil
- 1 teaspoon turmeric powder
- 1 large garlic clove, peeled and crushed
- 3 cm (1½ inch) knob fresh ginger, grated
- 1 large avocado, just ripe
- 2 limes, juiced
- 1 fresh ripe mango
- 2 large handfuls watercress, washed and roughly chopped
- Salt and freshly ground pepper
- 2 tablespoons coconut milk

1. Cook 100 g (3½ oz) of brown rice first using your favorite method.
2. In a bowl, mix the oil, turmeric, garlic and ginger together. Toss in the prawns and mix well. Allow them to sit in the marinade whilst you prepare the salad.
3. Slice the avocado in half lengthways. Quarter it lengthways, then remove the stone and skin. Chop the avocado into large bite sized pieces. Place in a salad bowl with the lime juice and gently mix.
4. Slice the mango on either side of the seed. Crisscross cut each piece of mango, then scoop mango cubes into the salad bowl.
5. Add the watercress and a pinch of salt and pepper. Do not mix together yet.
6. Warm a large frypan/skillet on medium heat, add the prawns and all the marinade and cook for 1–2 minutes on each side. Season with salt and pepper. Ensure they are cooked through to the center by cutting a large one. Add coconut milk to warm, then remove from the heat.
7. Toss the salad together gently.
8. Divide the warm cooked rice between two serving bowls, pile on the salad and top with the warm prawn mixture.

Note: Brazil nuts are also an excellent source of selenium (see Overnight Berry Oats recipe page 53).

Spicy Calamari with Okra, Avocado and Black Beans

Serves 2

Okra contains great fiber which helps to prevent and relieve constipation. This means our bodies can improve excretion of unwanted female hormones and toxins. Of course, there is fiber in many of the other ingredients in this recipe.

INGREDIENTS

Calamari
240 g (9 oz) squid or calamari, prepared for eating by the seafood supplier
1 tablespoon extra virgin olive oil
2 cloves garlic, peeled and finely chopped
1 long green chili, split, deseeded and finely chopped
1 big pinch salt
1 big pinch freshly ground pepper
1 teaspoon coriander (cilantro) powder
½ teaspoon smoked paprika (must be smoked)
2 teaspoons dried Greek oregano

Vegetables
3 tablespoons extra virgin olive oil
1 large red onion, finely sliced
175 g (6 oz) okra, washed and roughly sliced diagonally
200 g (7 oz) cherry tomatoes, washed
140 g (5 oz) cooked black beans (cook your own or canned)
Pinch salt and freshly ground pepper
2 tablespoons feta
½ lime, cut into 2 wedges
Handful coriander (cilantro) leaves, washed and chopped
½ large avocado flesh chopped into small pieces

1. Cut the calamari into large chunks or thick rings and toss with garlic, chili, salt, pepper, coriander, paprika and oregano and 1 tablespoon of oil. Leave marinating in the fridge whilst you cook the vegetables.
2. In a large frying pan/skillet add the 2 tablespoons of oil, okra and onions. Fry on medium heat, stirring frequently. Once the onions have softened, about 5 minutes, add the tomatoes.
3. Cook until the tomatoes begin to soften and break up. Then add the black beans to warm and add a pinch of salt and pepper.
4. Once warmed through, divide the vegetable and black beans onto 2 serving plates.
5. Wipe out the pan and heat on high, adding the calamari once the pan is hot.
6. Sear the calamari until it is just cooked and firmed up, about 1–2 minutes, stirring occasionally.
7. Place on top of the vegetables, squeeze over the lime juice, crumble over the feta, and scatter the coriander and avocado.

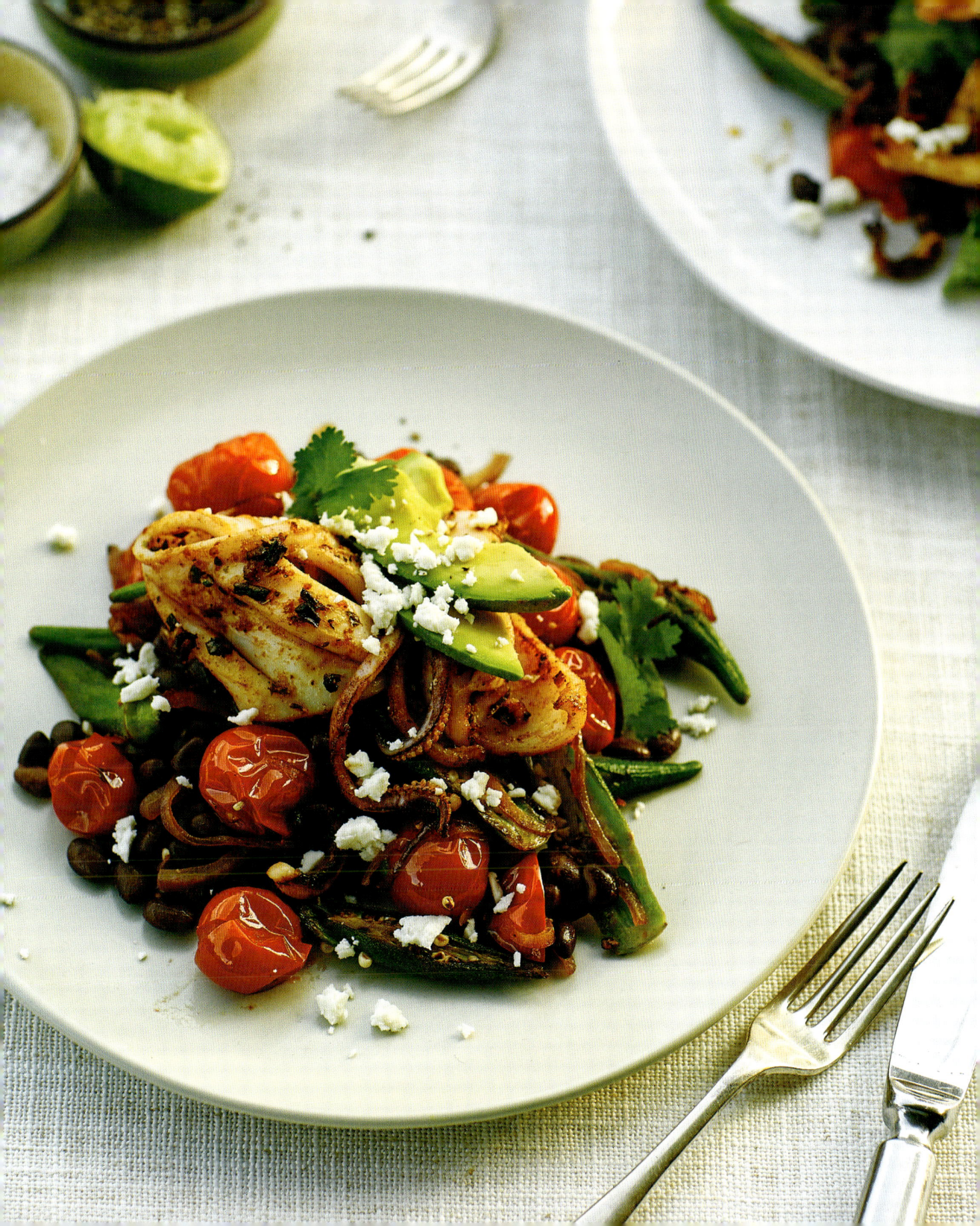

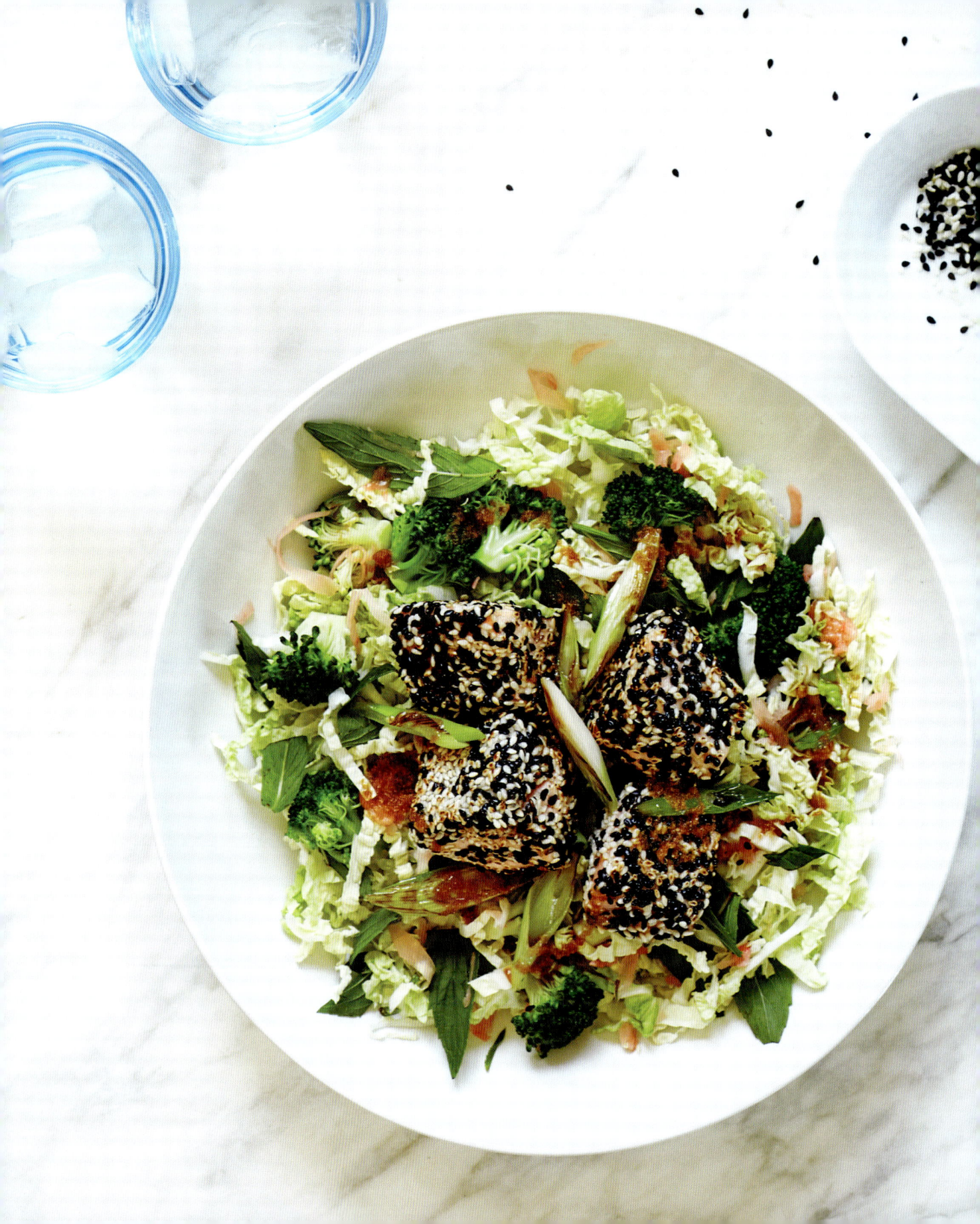

Sesame Crusted Salmon with Asian Slaw

Serves 2

Salmon is a great source of Omega 3 oils, which are beneficial for female hormone balance, both physically and emotionally, at any stage of a woman's life. Cabbage, broccoli and ginger are great for our liver.

INGREDIENTS

Salmon
220 g (8 oz) salmon fillet, cut into chunks about 4 cm (2 inch) square
2 tablespoons white and black sesame seeds
1 tablespoon coconut oil

Slaw
200 g (7 oz) broccoli, cut into very small florets
1 large handful fresh mint, washed and chopped
120 g (4½ oz) wombok (Chinese cabbage), very thinly sliced
4 spring onions (scallions), washed, roughly chopped by slicing diagonally
1 tablespoon thinly sliced pickled ginger (recipe page 35)

Dressing
1 tablespoon finely grated fresh ginger
1 heaped teaspoon miso paste
1 tablespoon rice vinegar
½–1 tablespoon Mirin
1 tablespoon tamari or soy sauce (tamari is wheat free)
1 tablespoon sesame oil

1. Mix all the dressing ingredients together, using a fork to smash the miso paste into the dressing.
2. Toss the salmon with the sesame seeds to roughly coat all over.
3. Blanch the broccoli in boiling water for about 2 minutes or steam for 4 minutes. Refresh in cold water to prevent the broccoli from cooking longer, then drain.
4. To a large frying pan/skillet or wok, on high heat, add the coconut oil and spring onions. Cook for about 30 seconds to just scorch the outside of the onions. Take them out of the pan.
5. Mix all the slaw ingredients together in a bowl. Don't add the dressing until just before serving, as the cabbage will wilt.
6. Add the salmon to the pan and sear on each side for about 30 seconds.
7. Toss the slaw with the dressing. Divide it between two plates and top with the seared salmon.

Roast Cauliflower with Mediterranean Salsa and Snapper

Serves 2

Bursting with phytonutrients, this dish helps to balance hormones, support liver function and reduce inflammation. The fish contains vitamin B6 and B12, both of which are used to help produce 'happy' neurotransmitter hormones in our bodies.

INGREDIENTS

Salad
500 g (17½ oz) of cauliflower cut into small florets
1 tablespoon extra virgin olive oil
Pinch of salt and freshly ground pepper
1 teaspoon cumin seeds
1 teaspoon fresh or dried thyme leaves
100 g (3½ oz) cooked chickpeas (cook your own or canned)

Salsa
1 tablespoon fresh lemon juice
5 cherry tomatoes, washed and diced
¼ long red chili, seeds removed and finely chopped
½ large ripe avocado, diced small
1 pickled anchovy fillet, finely chopped
30 g (1 oz) pitted black Kalamata olives
1 large handful basil leaves, washed and finely chopped
1 small clove garlic, peeled and crushed
1 heaped teaspoon baby capers
1 tablespoon extra virgin olive oil

Fish
250 g (9 oz) boneless snapper filets or other white fish
1 tablespoon extra virgin olive oil
Salt and pepper

1. Set your oven to 190°C (375°F) fan forced or 210°C (425°F) regular.
2. Toss the cauliflower in a bowl with oil, thyme, cumin, pepper and salt.
3. Place on a baking tray lined with baking/parchment paper. Make sure it is spread in one single layer. Put into the hot oven for 25–30 minutes.
4. In a separate bowl gently mix all the salsa ingredients together.
5. Rub salt, pepper and oil into your fish fillets. Lay on a baking tray lined with baking paper/parchment and put into the oven to roast for 10 minutes or until just cooked through.
6. Once the cauliflower has roasted for 25 minutes and is beginning to go brown at the edges, toss in the chickpeas to warm for the last 5 minutes of cooking.
7. Once everything is cooked and out of the oven, divide the cauliflower and chickpeas onto two plates, add the fish fillets and pour over any juices that remain. Top with the salsa.

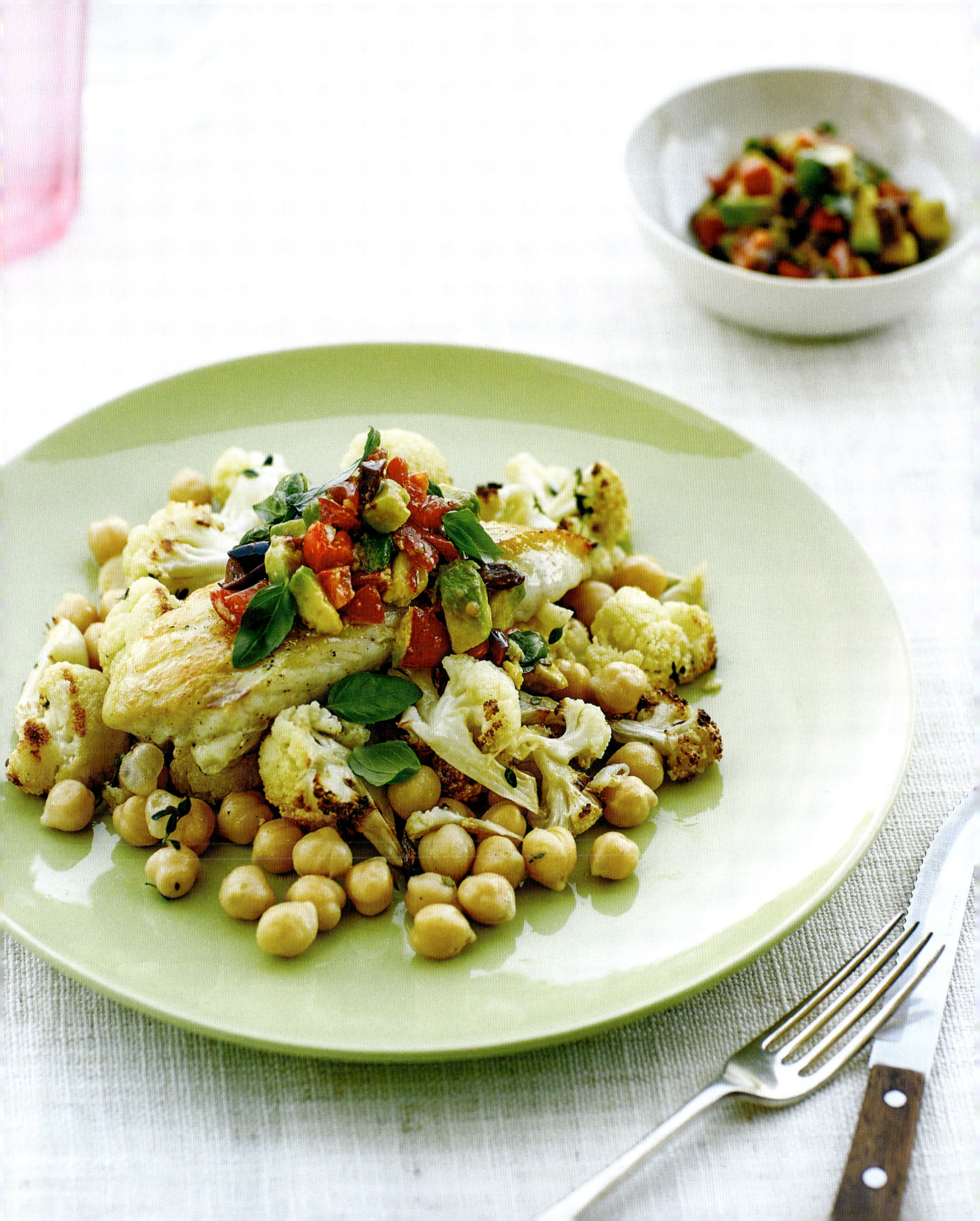

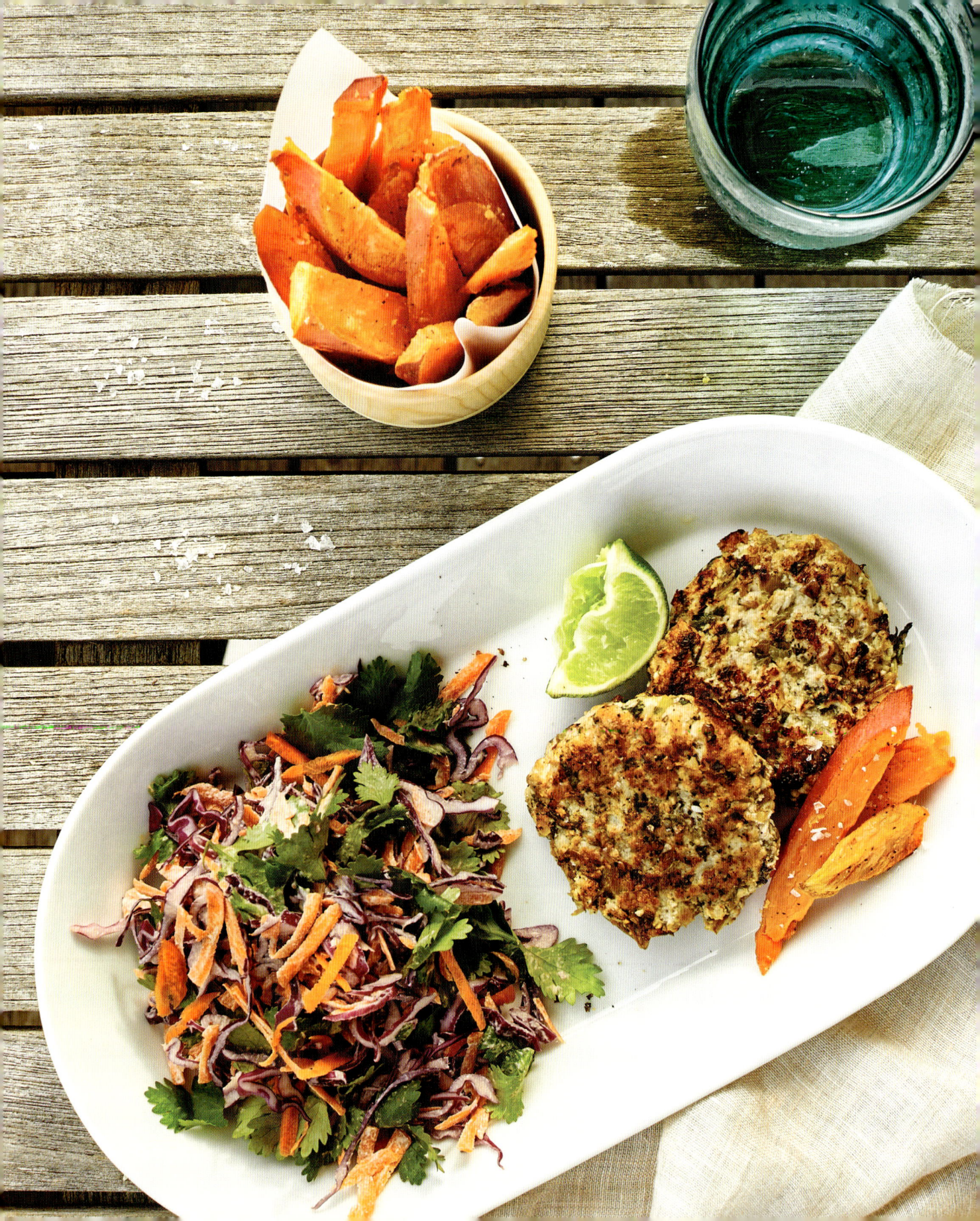

Fish Cakes with Sweet Potato Chips and Red Cabbage Slaw

Serves 4

The sweet potato in this dish is a really good source of vitamin B6. B6 is required for hormone production and helps relieve the symptoms of PMS and menopause including mood, pain and depression. The Omega 3 oils in the fish add further help with these symptoms.

Sweet potato is also high in beta-carotene, which converts to vitamin A. This is used in our bodies for mucus membrane support and tissue repair in female reproductive organs.

INGREDIENTS

Fish Cakes
- 1 big handful basil leaves, washed
- 2 large spring onions (scallions) roughly chopped
- 1 tablespoon capers, rinsed
- Zest and juice of 1 large lemon
- 1 long green chili, deseeded and roughly chopped
- 4 tablespoons cooked red lentils (either freshly cooked or canned)
- Big pinch of salt and freshly ground pepper
- 400 g (14 oz) boneless fish fillets, such as salmon

Chips
- 1 unpeeled (550 g (18 oz)) sweet potato (kumara), washed
- A big pinch of salt and freshly ground pepper
- 1 tablespoon extra virgin olive oil

Slaw
- ¼ (150 g (5 oz)) red cabbage, finely sliced
- 2 large carrots, grated
- 1 handful washed coriander (cilantro) leaves

Dressing
- 2 tablespoons tahini
- 2 tablespoons unsweetened natural organic yogurt (not coconut)

1. Heat your oven to 200°C (390°F) fan forced or 220°C (430°F) regular.
2. Cut the sweet potato into chips or wedges. Toss in a bowl with olive oil, salt and pepper.
3. Line a baking tray with oven/parchment paper and spread the chips onto this so they form one layer. Place the potato in the oven to bake for 40 minutes or until it is cooked and crispy on the outside. Every 15 minutes take the tray out of the oven and loosen the chips before putting them back into the oven.
4. Put all the fish cake ingredients, except the fish, into a food processor and blend until well ground – approximately 1 minute. Scrape down the sides and blend a little more.
5. Then add the fish fillets. Pulse for about 5 seconds to chop up the fish. Do not make a paste of it. However, make sure it is mixed through.
6. Oil your hands and roll out 4 large fish cakes from the mixture. Put them into an ovenproof frying pan/skillet and fry on one side for 1 minute. Then carefully turn them over and place the pan in the oven to bake for a further 10 minutes or until they are cooked all the way through.
7. Mix the yogurt with the tahini. Toss through the cabbage, carrot and coriander. Check the taste and add a pinch of salt and pepper, if you think it needs it.
8. Put the slaw into a salad bowl.
9. Once the chips are cooked, put them into a serving dish and serve the fish cakes on individual plates.

Wombok, Asparagus and Mushroom Salad with Salmon
Serves 2

There are so many excellent nutrients in this dish for female hormone balance.
- Omega 3 anti-inflammatory oils in the salmon
- Great liver phytonutrients in the vegetables
- Calcium in the cabbage, seeds, herbs, seaweed, asparagus and spinach

There's plenty of flavor and it takes very little time to cook!

INGREDIENTS

- 240 g (9 oz) raw salmon fillet
- 2 tablespoons extra virgin olive oil or coconut oil
- 2 teaspoons sesame oil
- 1 bunch asparagus spears
- 100 g (3 ½ oz) mushrooms, preferably Asian style mushrooms, such as shiitake.
- 150 g (5 oz) wombok (Chinese cabbage), finely shredded
- 2 spring onions (scallions), washed and thinly sliced
- 2 handfuls spinach leaves, washed
- A handful mint leaves, washed
- 1 tablespoon fresh ginger, grated
- ½ bunch coriander (cilantro), well washed
- 2 tablespoons sesame seeds
- 1 sheet of Nori (the seaweed sheets used to wrap sushi)
- ½ lime, cut into 2 wedges
- Soy sauce or tamari

1. Slice the salmon fillet into small slices about 1 cm (½ inch) thick, leaving the skin on if you wish.
2. In a wok or large frying pan/skillet put 1 tablespoon of oil and sesame seeds. Don't heat yet.
3. Wash and break the woody end off the asparagus. Then cut them in half and slice again lengthways. Add to the wok.
4. Slice the mushrooms and put into the wok along with the spinach, Chinese cabbage, mint, ginger and spring onions.
5. Chop off the leaves of the coriander. Then finely chop the coriander stalks and roots, and add to the wok.
6. Using kitchen scissors thinly cut the Nori sheet into the vegetables in the wok.
7. Turn the wok heat to high and stir fry its contents for about 1–2 minutes, so that the spinach leaves are just wilted. Divide between two serving plates.
8. Drizzle the sesame oil onto the vegetables.
9. Wipe out the same wok or frying pan and add another tablespoon oil. Put in the salmon pieces and sear for 15 seconds each side.
10. Place the salmon on top of the vegetables. Squeeze over the lime juice and drizzle some soy or tamari sauce to taste.

Black Bean and Mushroom Stew (V)

Serves 2

A delicious stew! The fiber in black beans is particularly beneficial for the healthy bacteria in our gut, allowing these bacteria to produce butyrate (see Gut Health page 18). Black beans also contain many of the nutrients we need to maintain bone health. The black color is where most of the phytonutrients are, particularly anthocyanins, which have both antioxidant and anti-inflammatory roles. They help our cells to withstand stress.

INGREDIENTS

- 400 g (14 oz) sweet potato (kumara), washed, unpeeled and roughly chopped
- 25 g (1 oz) almonds
- 2 tablespoons extra virgin olive oil
- 1 bay leaf
- 1 teaspoon smoked paprika (must be smoked)
- 2 heaped teaspoons ground cumin
- 100 g (3½ oz) small red onion, finely chopped
- 2 garlic cloves, peeled and crushed
- ½ bunch coriander (cilantro)
- 1 long red chili or 1 teaspoon dried chili flakes
- 100 g (3½ oz) cherry tomatoes, roughly chopped
- ½ red capsicum, washed, deseeded and chopped into bite-size pieces
- 150 g (5 oz) cooked black beans (cook your own or canned)
- 125 ml (4 fl oz) black bean cooking liquid, vegetable stock or water
- 2 large field mushrooms
- Salt and freshly ground pepper
- 2 heaped tablespoons natural unsweetened yogurt
- ½ lime

1. Steam the sweet potato until soft, about 15–20 minutes.
2. Roughly chop the almonds and, in a large dry frying pan/skillet, toast them on medium heat for about 1 minute.
3. Tip the almonds into a small bowl and wipe the pan clean, putting it back on the stove.
4. Put the olive oil, bay leaf, paprika and cumin into the pan. Warm on a low to moderate heat for about a minute.
5. Add the onion and garlic to the pan and soften, about 4 minutes.
6. Wash the coriander, removing any grit from the roots and stalks. Cut off the leaves and reserve for later. Finely cut up the roots and stalks and add to the onions.
7. Slice the chili lengthways and scrape out the seeds. Finely chop and add to the onion mix. (Use less chili if you're not such a fan. Leave the seeds in, if you like it hot.)
8. Add the tomatoes and capsicum to the mix. Cook everything slowly for about 5–7 minutes.
9. Add the black beans and their liquid and stir to warm.
10. Thickly slice the field mushrooms and add them to the pan, covering them well with the liquid. Allow them to cook until soft, about 5 minutes. They will absorb some of the delicious sauce.
11. Season the stew with salt and pepper to taste.
12. Once the sweet potato is cooked, mash it, adding salt and pepper to taste.
13. To serve, divide the sweet potato mash into two large shallow bowls. Then divide the mushroom stew between the two. Dollop a heaped tablespoon of yogurt. Scatter the almonds and chopped coriander leaves over the top. Add a squeeze of lime juice.

Harissa-crusted Mushrooms with Lentil, Pomegranate and Eggplant (V)

Serves 2

This is a delicious vegetarian dish, which provides plenty of antioxidant phytonutrients. The lentils help the liver to process unwanted female hormones and toxins. Lentils also aid the movement of food through our digestive system, helping to prevent constipation. The fiber in this dish feeds our beneficial gut bacteria, which means our gut is likely to make more of the 'happy' hormone, serotonin.

INGREDIENTS

- 1 eggplant (aubergine), washed
- 2 tablespoons extra virgin olive oil, plus 1 tablespoon for brushing eggplant
- 2–3 teaspoons Harrisa paste
- 4 large field mushrooms
- Big pinch salt and freshly ground pepper
- 130 g (4½ oz) cooked black Lentils (cook your own or canned)
- 1 pomegranate, cut in half with seeds tapped out, aim for 100 g (3½ oz) of pomegranate seeds
- Large handful parsley, washed and finely chopped
- 20 g (1 oz) shelled pistachios, roughly chopped

Dressing
- 2 tablespoons natural unsweetened yogurt
- 2 tablespoons tahini paste
- 1 teaspoon cumin powder
- ½ lemon or 1 large lime, juiced

1. You can cook this dish on the BBQ, under the grill or in your oven on 180°C (350°F) fan forced of 200°C (390°F) regular.
2. Cut the eggplant into 2.5 cm (1 inch) slices and brush with olive oil on both sides of each slice. Place them under the grill or on BBQ, turning over once the first side has gone slightly golden brown. If cooking in the oven, bake for 20–25 minutes. Cook until they feel soft in the center, then let them rest on a plate.
3. Mix the Harrisa paste with 2 tablespoons of oil. If you like your mushrooms chili-hot, then add another teaspoon of paste.
4. Brush the mushrooms with the paste and sprinkle over salt and pepper. Cook on the BBQ, under the grill or in the oven until they are just soft, about 8 minutes, if you are cooking in the oven.
5. In a bowl mix the dressing ingredients together with a fork.
6. Roughly chop the eggplant into large bite sized pieces, toss into the bowl with the lentils, pomegranate, parsley and some of the pistachios. Then massage the dressing through.
7. Divide onto 2 serving plates.
8. Thickly slice the mushrooms, place on top and sprinkle with the remaining pistachios.

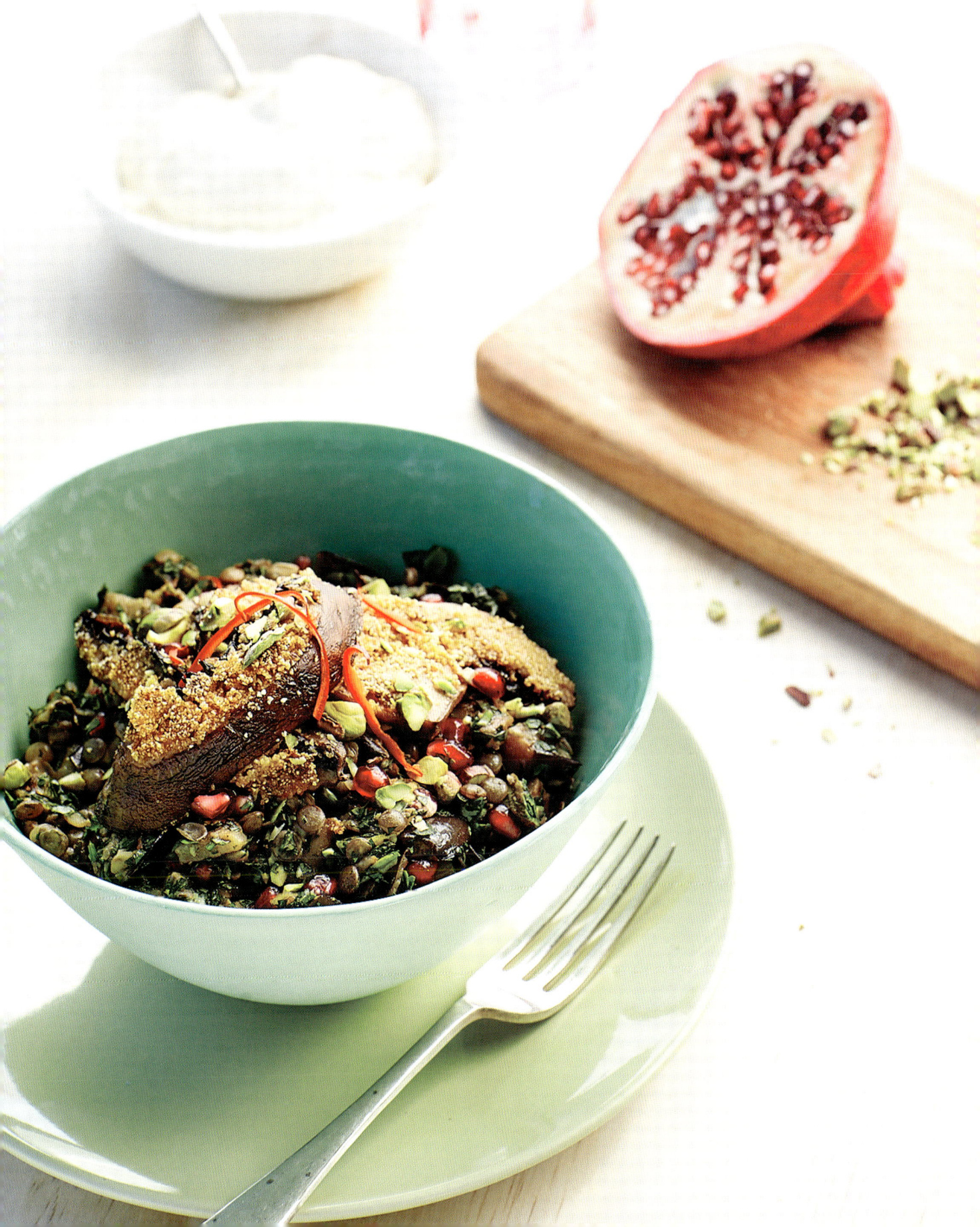

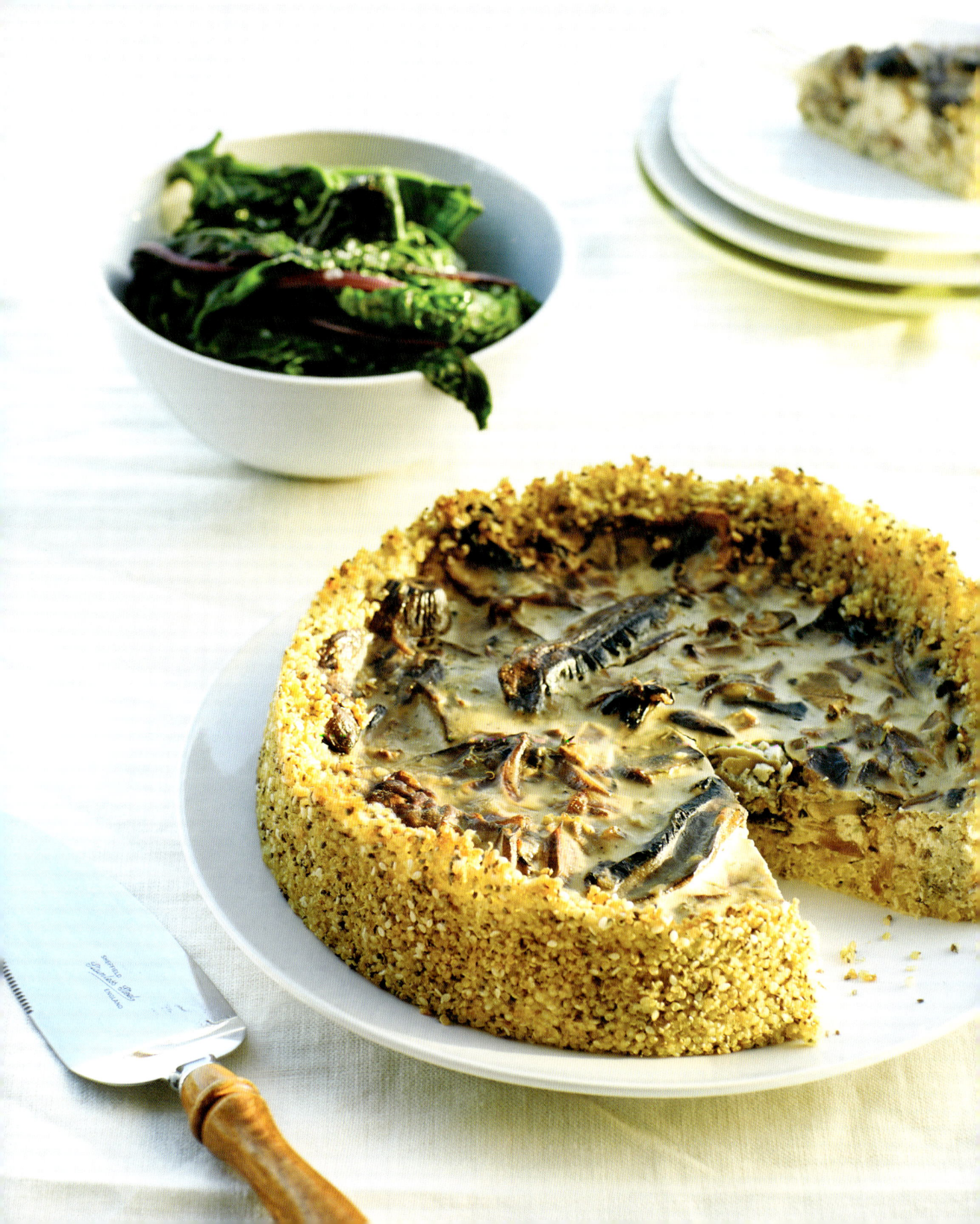

Quinoa Crusted Mushroom Pie with Wilted Greens (V)

Pie serves 6–8/ Wilted greens serve 4

Sometimes it is fun to have a pie! The abundance of mushrooms in this pie helps to support our immune system and reduce inflammation, so female organs and hormone production can be enhanced. They also contain B vitamins helpful in energy production. Any leftovers can be cut into wedges and eaten as lunch or a snack.

INGREDIENTS

Crust
- 600 g (22 oz) well cooked quinoa, any color
- 2 tablespoons sesame seeds
- 2 tablespoons black chia seeds
- 1 heaped tablespoon freshly grated parmesan cheese (optional)
- 1 large organic free range egg, lightly beaten
- Big pinch of salt and freshly ground pepper

Filling
- 3 large organic free range eggs, lightly beaten
- 280 g (9½ oz) goat, sheep, buffalo or cow's yogurt (not thickened)
- Salt and freshly ground white pepper
- 1 tablespoon extra virgin olive oil
- 1 large red onion, finely chopped
- 450 g (16 oz) large field mushrooms, sliced mushrooms
- 15 g (1 oz) dried porcini mushrooms
- 1 large clove of garlic, peeled and crushed
- 1 heaped tablespoon fresh thyme leaves or tarragon or basil. Use dried if you don't have fresh
- 25 g (1 oz) freshly grated Parmesan cheese, blue or other hard cheese

Greens
- 2 teaspoons extra virgin olive oil
- 1 bunch spinach or ½ bunch silverbeet, kale or Swiss chard, washed and roughly chopped
- ½ lemon

1. Set your oven to 180°C (350°F) fan forced or 200°C (400°F) regular.
2. Cook 200 g (7 oz) of raw quinoa first.
3. Lightly oil a 22 cm (8 ½ inch) diameter springform cake tin. Line the bottom and sides with baking/parchment paper.
4. Soak the porcini mushrooms in warm water for 10 minutes, then drain and roughly chop them.
5. Mix the crust ingredients together and thinly press all around the tin. Begin with the sides, then fill the base, pressing firmly to ensure the crust sticks.
6. Mix the eggs, yogurt, salt and pepper in a large bowl, and leave to one side.
7. Gently fry the onion and mushrooms in a pan on a low heat until soft, about 5 minutes. Take off the heat and tip into a bowl to cool. Add the garlic, thyme and cheese, plus a big pinch of salt and pepper. Stir well, then tip into the egg mix and stir through.
8. Pour this mixture into the crust-lined cake tin. Place in the oven to bake for about 40 minutes, until the egg is only just cooked.
9. Rest for about 10 minutes out of the oven before cutting.
10. Wilt the greens in a pan with the olive oil and a good pinch of salt and pepper. Squeeze over the lemon juice and serve with the pie.

Oh-so-slow-cooked Beef with Sweet Potato • Serves 4

Beef is a great source of heme iron, the iron most easily absorbed by our bodies.

The beef in this dish is an inexpensive cut. By cooking it slowly the beef becomes more easily digestible, which enables our bodies to take more of the nutrients from it. It also becomes tender and is really delicious.

The Massaman Curry Paste can be time consuming to make. If you don't want to make your own, then buy a good quality one.

INGREDIENTS

Massaman Paste
1 bunch coriander (cilantro), washed well
1 lemongrass stem
2.5 cm (1 inch) knob ginger, washed but not peeled, roughly chopped
1 teaspoon cumin seeds
2 heaped teaspoons coriander (cilantro) seeds
½ teaspoon nutmeg powder
½ teaspoon cinnamon powder
½ teaspoon cloves powder
2 teaspoons turmeric powder
4 kaffir lime leaves, roughly chopped
2 teaspoons salt
1 teaspoon freshly ground pepper
1 tablespoon fish sauce
2 large long red chilis including seeds, roughly chopped

Curry
4 spring onions (scallions), washed and roughly chopped
1 tablespoon coconut oil
500 g (17½ oz) beef chuck, gravy beef or goat meat
500 g (17½ oz) sweet potato (kumara), washed (no need to peel)
2 whole kaffir lime leaves
Leftover lemongrass husks
3 whole star anise cloves
400 ml (13 fl oz) coconut milk

Garnish
4 large handful of spinach or kale, washed and chopped
1 large lime, cut into quarters
400 g (14 oz) cooked brown rice

1. You will need a slow cooker or a casserole dish with a lid for this recipe. If using a casserole dish, set your oven to 150°C (300°F) fan forced or 170°C (325°F) regular.

To make Massaman Paste:
1. Cut 1.5 cm (½ inch) off the bottom and at least half of the top off the lemongrass and save for the curry. From the remaining piece, pull away any woody layers and keep. Roughly chop the remainder.
2. Chop the roots and lower half of stems of the coriander and save the leaves to use later.
3. Blend all the paste ingredients in a small grinder or mortar and pestle until paste-like.

To make Curry:
1. Cut the meat and the sweet potato into chunks about 4 cm x 4 cm (1.5 inch x 1.5 inch).
2. Put the Massaman paste and oil into a large casserole dish on the stove on medium heat or in the slow cooker set on sauté. Fry off the paste for a couple of minutes, then add the onions. Cook for another minute.
3. Add the meat, searing the beef for about 4 minutes on all sides. Mix it well with the spices.
4. Then mix in all the other ingredients really well.
5. Put the lid on and cook in the oven or slow cooker for 4 hours, or follow the slow cooker instructions.
6. Once cooked and ready to serve, check if it needs any extra salt.
7. 30 minutes before your curry is ready, cook the brown rice.
8. Place hot cooked brown rice in each serving bowl. Add a handful of greens to each, to wilt under the heat of the curry. Spoon in a portion of the curry and squeeze the lime over the top.

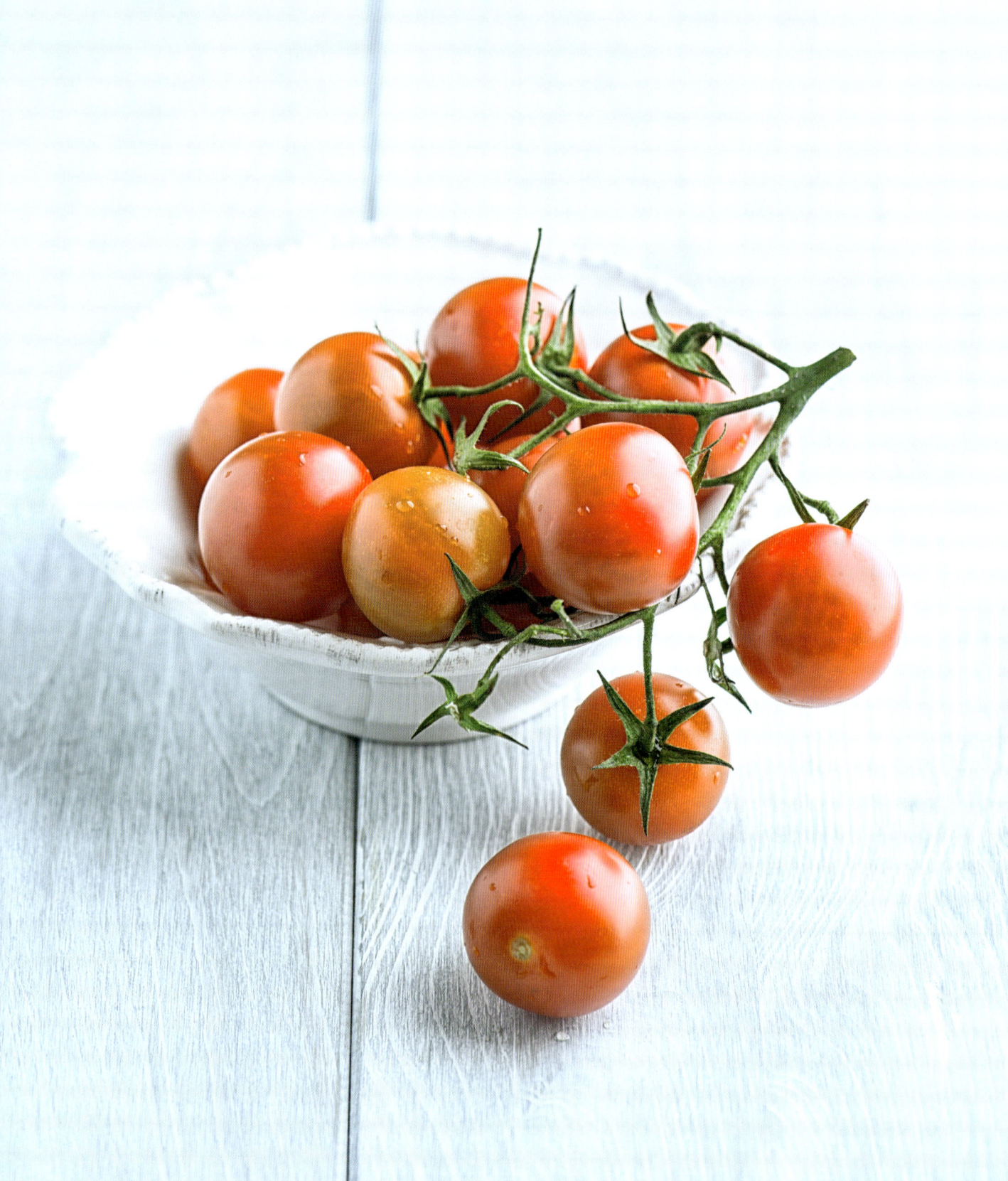

Baked Vegetables with Smokey Paprika (V)

Serves 2

This is a lovely way to increase your vegetable and phytonutrient intake. The broad beans are a prebiotic food and have phytoestrogen benefits (Fiber see page 15). The prebiotic food encourages our beneficial gut bacteria to aid the body's production of serotonin, one of the 'happy' hormones.

INGREDIENTS

- 1 small sweet potato (kumara), washed
- 400 g (14 oz) eggplant (aubergine), washed
- 1 large red onion, peeled
- 4 cloves garlic, peeled and crushed
- 3 green zucchini (courgettes), washed
- 3 tablespoons extra virgin olive oil
- Big pinch salt and freshly ground pepper
- 1 punnet cherry tomatoes, washed
- 250 g (9 oz) fresh or frozen broad (fava) beans
- 1 teaspoon smoked paprika (must be smoked)
- 25 g (1 oz) pepitas
- 25 g (1 oz) sunflower seeds

Optional: For non-vegetarian eaters you can add 120 g (4½ oz) of cooked chicken, beef or fish, per person.

1. Set your oven to 180°C (350°F) fan forced or 200°C (390°F) regular.
2. Chop the sweet potato into small bite size pieces and roughly chop the eggplant, onion and zucchini into large bite size pieces.
3. In a large bowl toss the sweet potato, eggplant, onion, garlic and zucchini together with 2 tablespoons of olive oil, salt and pepper.
4. Tip onto a large baking tray lined with baking/parchment paper. Spread out into a single layer, put into the oven and bake for 25 minutes.
5. After 15 minutes, scatter the tomatoes over the top of the vegetables.
6. Cook the broad (fava) beans in boiling water for 2 minutes if frozen or for 3 minutes if fresh. Drain, then plunge them into cold water to refresh and drain.
7. If you wish, peel the skins off the beans. If your beans are young and fresh or smallish and are a good quality frozen brand, this is not necessary. It's personal taste.
8. Toss the pepitas and sunflower seeds with the paprika and 1 tablespoon olive oil and add to the baking vegetables once they have cooked for 25 minutes. Cook for a further 5 minutes.
9. Remove from the oven and cool to touch.
10. Place the vegetable mix into a large bowl, add the cooked beans and mix together ensuring the paprika coats the vegetables. The tomatoes may break up a bit, creating a sauce. This is fine.
11. Check the seasoning and add more salt and pepper, if required.
12. Divide the vegetables between the two serving plates and toss through shredded chicken, beef or fish, if desired.

Parsley and Quinoa Tabouli with Lamb

Serves 2, with leftovers of tabouli

Lamb is a great source of iron, a mineral needed by women, and often lower in women than men, due to a combination of diets low in iron and menstrual blood loss. The parsley, high in vitamin C contains its own form of non-heme iron, which helps the body absorb the iron. In fact, the presence of heme iron in the lamb enhances the absorption of the non-heme iron in the parsley.

INGREDIENTS

Lamb
240 g (9 oz) lamb backstrap or lamb fillets
1 heaped teaspoon ground coriander (cilantro)
1 heaped teaspoon ground cumin
1 teaspoon dried thyme
Big pinch of cayenne pepper
1 tablespoon extra virgin olive oil

Tabouli
200 g (7 oz) white quinoa, cooked
1 tablespoon extra virgin olive oil, plus extra for brushing eggplant
300 g (10½ oz) eggplant (aubergine), washed
Pinch salt and freshly ground pepper
2 handfuls mint leaves, washed
2 handfuls flat leaf (continental) parsley leaves, washed
35 g (1 oz) almonds
25 g (1 oz) pistachio nuts
2 spring onions (scallions), washed and finely chopped
1 clove garlic, peeled and crushed
130 g (4½ oz) cherry tomatoes, washed and finely diced
1 lemon
80 g (3 oz) hummus (recipe page 184)

Continued on page 127

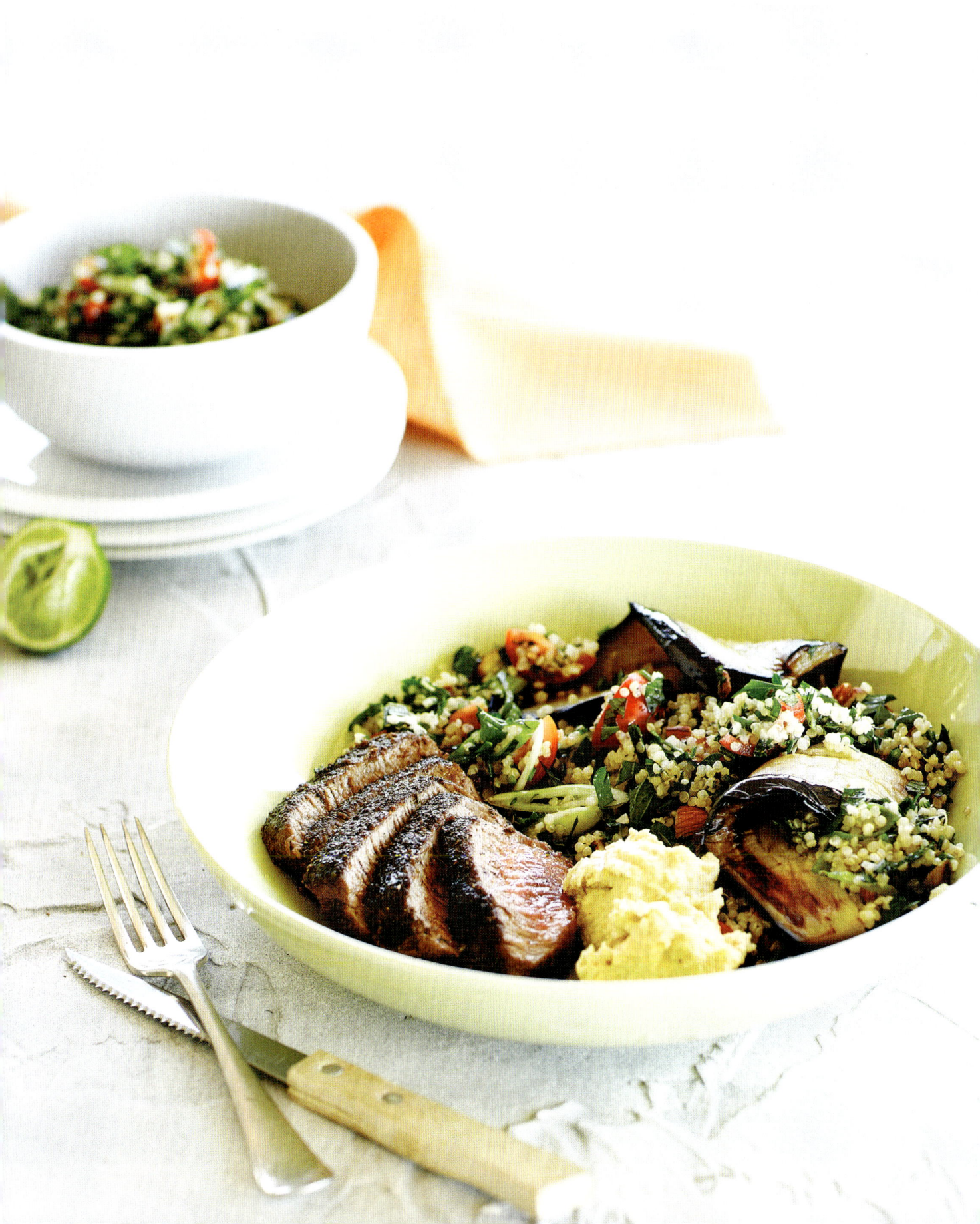

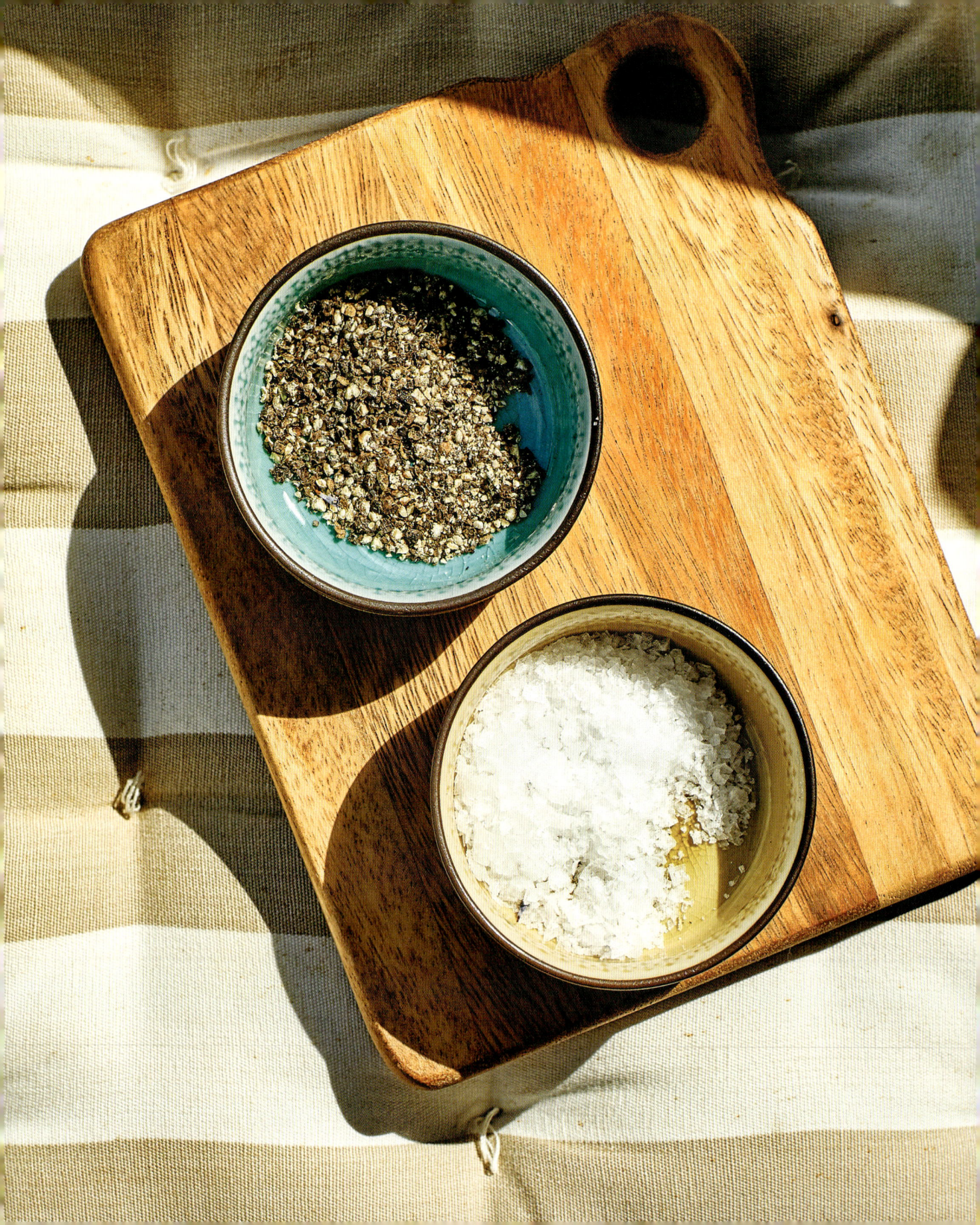

1. Set your oven to 180°C (350°F) fan forced or 200°C (400°F) regular oven. Alternatively, heat your BBQ or grill on medium.

To make Lamb:
1. Mix the spices and olive oil together in a bowl, add the lamb and coat really well. Leave to marinate in the fridge overnight or for an hour or two.

To make Tabouli:
1. Cook 100 g (3 ½ oz) of quinoa as per the packet instructions. Once cooked, allow it to cool.
2. Cut the eggplant into slices 1 cm (½ inch) thick. Lightly brush with olive oil, season with a little salt and pepper and place in a single layer on a baking tray lined with baking/parchment paper. Put into the oven and bake for about 20 minutes or until soft.
3. Roughly chop the parsley and mint leaves. Put them into a mixing bowl along with the cooled quinoa.
4. Roughly chop the almonds and pistachios and toast them in a dry frying pan/skillet for a couple of minutes on medium heat. Keep them moving around the pan and watch they don't catch and burn. Tip ¾ of them into the quinoa mix. Save the rest to scatter on top at the end.
5. Add the spring onions, garlic and tomatoes to the quinoa plus the juice from half the lemon and 1 tablespoon of oil. Season with salt and pepper and toss together.
6. Wipe out the pan. Put it back on the stove on medium heat and sear the lamb for 30 seconds on each side. Then put it into the oven for 5 minutes. Because lamb backstrap is lean, it cooks quickly and will dry out if over cooked. Take out of the oven and rest for 5–10 minutes before cutting. It should still be pink in the middle.
7. Meanwhile take the eggplant out of the oven and divide between two serving plates.
8. Dollop the hummus on the eggplant and spoon the quinoa tabouli on top.
9. Once the lamb has rested, thickly slice it and place on the tabouli. Squeeze over the remaining lemon and serve

Note: As an alternative to lamb, you can use venison or kangaroo fillets.

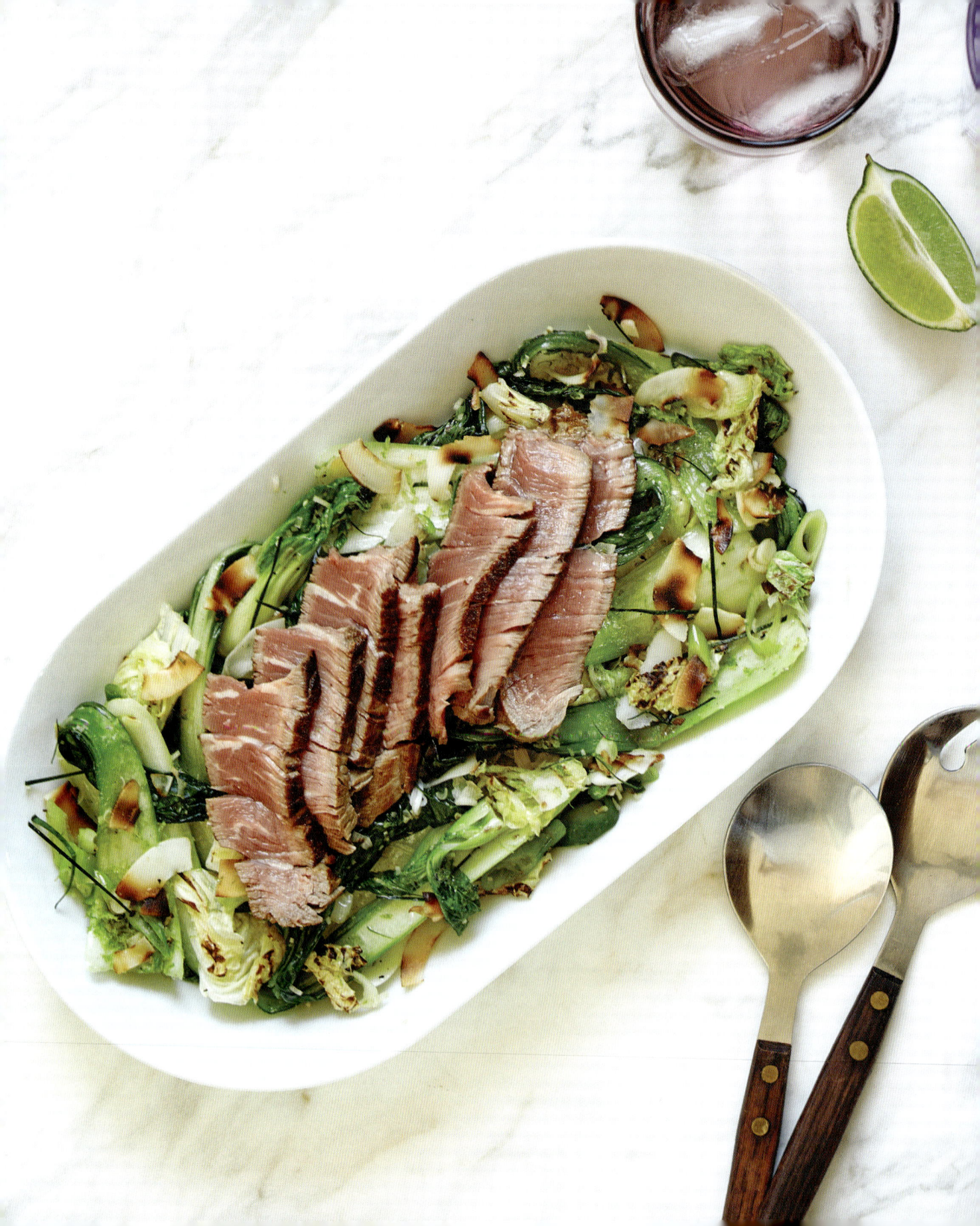

Seared Beef with Lime, Lemongrass and Coconut Salad

Serves 2

Organic beef provides a great source of heme iron; the iron most easily absorbed into our bodies. You only need a small quantity of beef to achieve this. The bok choy, onions and cabbage all help to support the liver's detoxification process of unwanted female hormones and toxins.

INGREDIENTS

Salad
- 2 small beef steaks, about 130 g (4½ oz) each
- Salt and freshly ground pepper
- 1 bunch bok choy or Pak Choy, washed
- 1 tablespoon extra virgin olive oil
- 2 large spring onions (scallions), washed and finely chopped
- 1 handful unsweetened coconut chips
- 1 long green chili, seeds removed and finely sliced
- 100 g (3½ oz) wombok (Chinese cabbage), cut into large bite-size pieces
- 1 lemongrass stalk
- 4 fresh kaffir lime leaves, stalk removed and very finely chopped
- Zest of 2 limes

Dressing
- Juice from 2 limes
- ½ tablespoon fish sauce
- 1 tablespoon extra virgin olive oil
- ½ teaspoon honey

1. Cut the bottom 2 cm (1 inch) and half the top off the lemongrass stalk. Remove the outer fibrous husks until you get to the softer flesh. Finely chop this, removing any husk still remaining as you cut.
2. Sear two beef fillets on medium heat in a frying pan/skillet, so they are cooked rare. Season with a pinch of salt and a big grind of pepper as you cook them. Then leave to rest on a plate and wipe clean the frying pan.
3. Cut the white bulb and stalks cut off the bok choy and discard. Toss the leaves into a bowl with 1 tablespoon oil and a pinch of salt and pepper. Put into a frying pan, on medium heat, and toss the bok choy, scorching the leaves, until they have just wilted, about 1 minute. Remove from the pan and put into your salad bowl.
4. Toss the spring onions, coconut chips and green chili in the hot pan. Scorch for about 1 minute and then tip into the salad bowl.
5. Scorch the wombok for 1 minute in the pan and toss into the bowl.
6. Add the lemongrass, kaffir lime leaves and lime zest to your bowl.
7. To make dressing: Squeeze the juice from both limes into a small bowl. Add the fish sauce, honey and sesame oil. Mix together and pour over the salad. Toss together and divide onto 2 serving plates.
8. Finely slice the meat and place on top of each of the salad.

Note: Kangaroo fillets are a great alternative to beef. Or, if you have any leftover meat from the previous day, it can be shredded and added into the salad instead of the beef.

Roast Pumpkin and Olive Salad with Haloumi (V)

Serves 4

This salad contains great fiber for our gut, in the following:
- Pumpkin (especially in the skin)
- Asparagus (especially prebiotic inulin fiber)
- Lentils (especially soluble fiber which 'grabs' bile and any excess or toxic hormones contained in the bile)

Pumpkin also contains an excellent supply of B vitamins, used in energy production and blood sugar regulation in our bodies.

INGREDIENTS
500 g (17½ oz) raw pumpkin with skin on
3 tablespoons extra virgin olive oil
Big pinch salt and freshly ground pepper
6 fat asparagus spears
1 teaspoon cumin seeds
40 g (1½ oz) walnuts
50 g (2 oz) black Kalamata olives, pitted
200 g (7 oz) lentils, sprouted or cooked
85 g (3 oz) rocket leaves
3 tablespoons lemon juice
250 g (9 oz) Haloumi cheese, preferably organic

---

1. Set your oven to 180°C (350°F) fan-forced or 200°C (400°F) regular.
2. Wash and then cut the pumpkin into thin wedges, no need to peel or deseed.
3. Toss the pumpkin wedges in a big bowl with 1 tablespoon of oil, salt and pepper. Place the pumpkin in a single layer on a large baking tray with baking/parchment paper. Then pull the pumpkin seeds away from the pumpkin flesh and spread out to back on the tray. Roast in the hot oven for 15 minutes.
4. Carefully wash the asparagus spears and break off the woody end (usually the lower ⅓ of the stem). Cut the remaining spear in half.
5. Put the asparagus and cumin seeds into the bowl you used to toss the pumpkin. Toss around in the residue of oil. Add in a little more salt and pepper, if you wish.
6. Once the pumpkin has cooked for 15 minutes, add the asparagus and cumin mix to the pumpkin tray to roast for a further 5 minutes. Take out of the oven to cool.
7. Roughly chop the walnuts and olives and put into the mixing bowl (no need to wash it out).
8. Add lentils, rocket and lemon juice, plus 2 tablespoons of oil.
9. Add ¼ teaspoon salt and ¼ teaspoon ground pepper, and the cooled pumpkin and asparagus. Using your hands, gently toss together.
10. Slice the Haloumi into 1 cm (½ inch) thick slices. On medium heat, fry them in a frying pan/skillet, on both sides (about 1–2 minutes each side) until soft. You may need a little olive oil to stop the Haloumi from sticking.
11. Spoon the salad onto serving plates and top with the Haloumi.

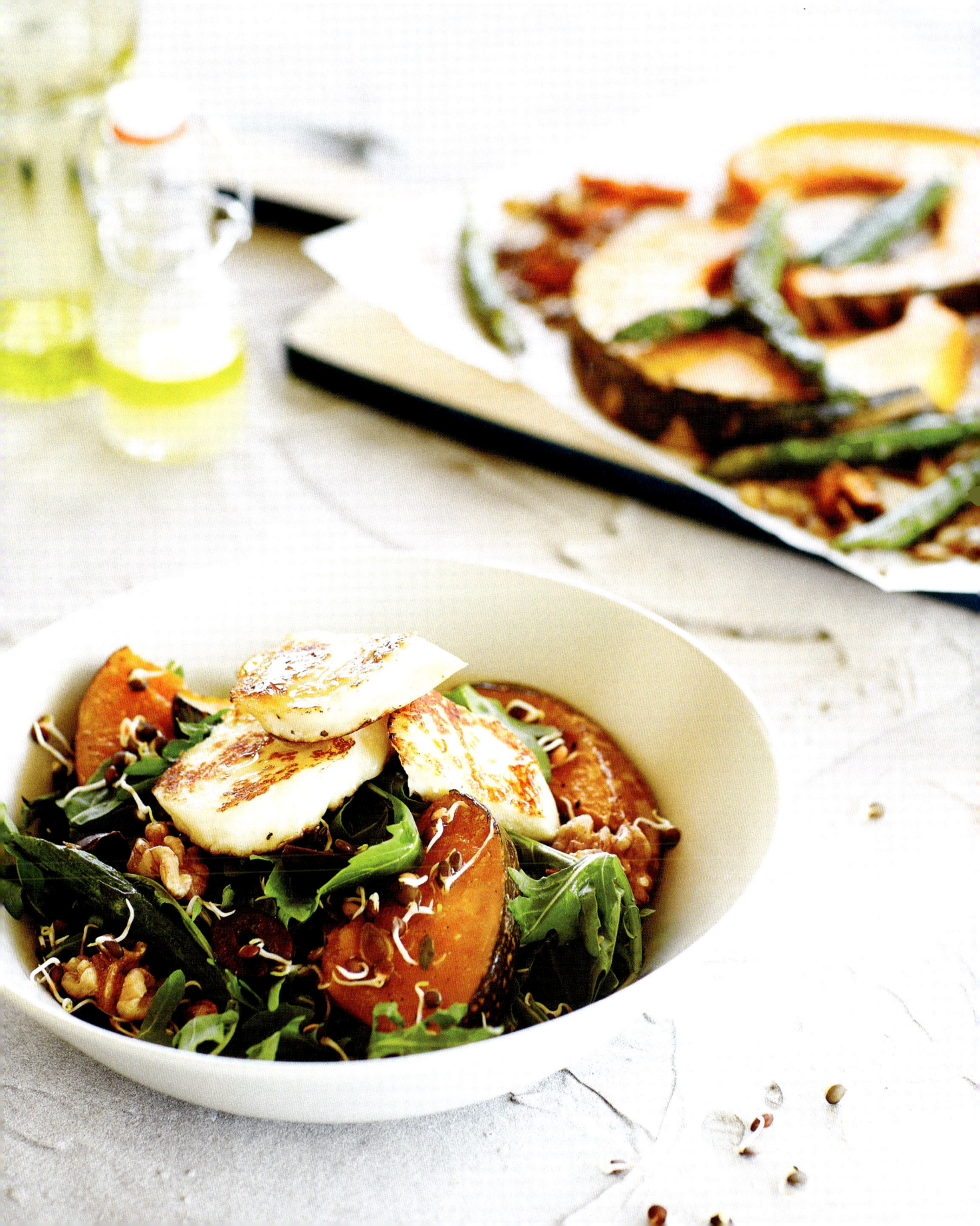

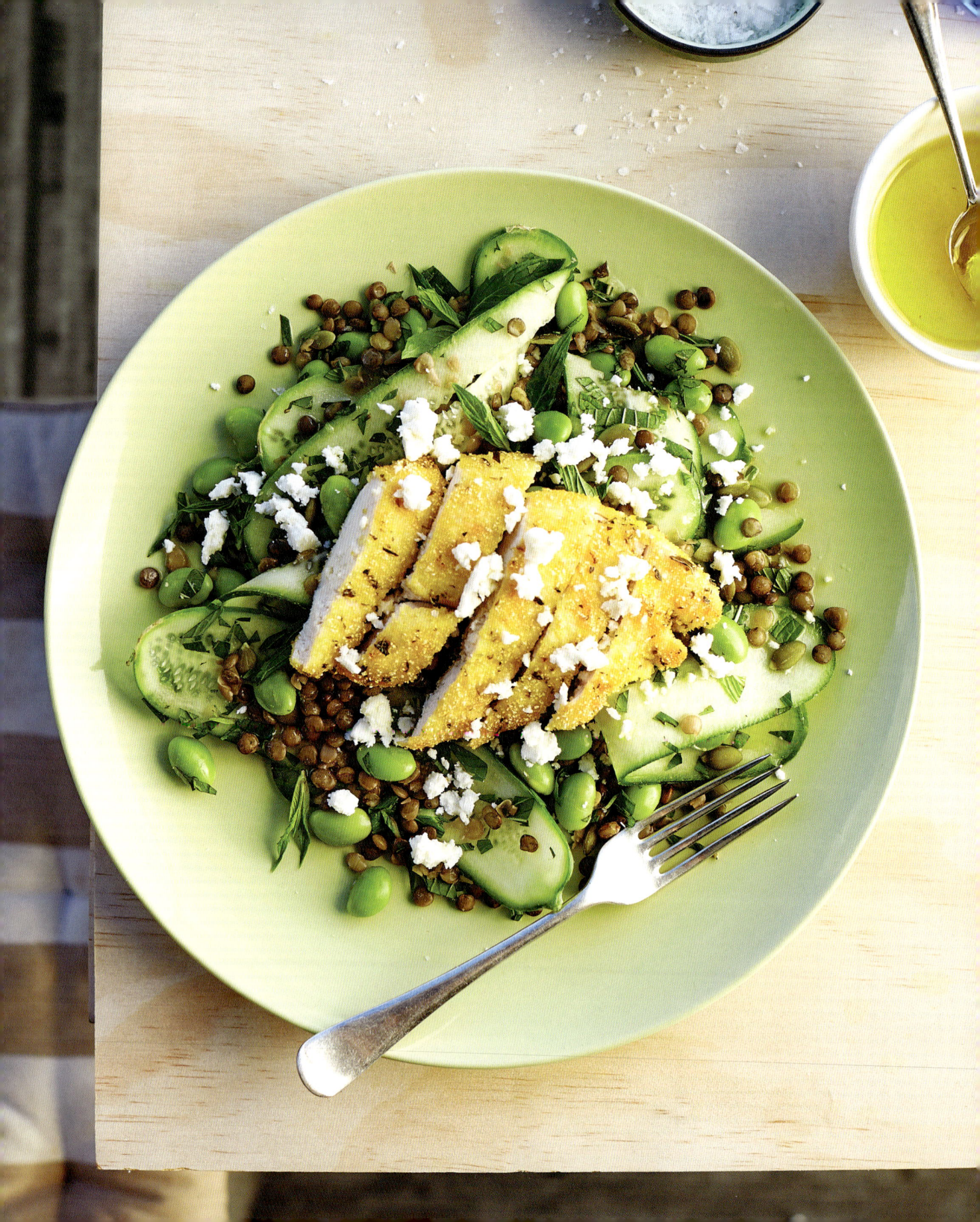

Mint and Bean Salad with Polenta Chicken

Serves 4

This is a tasty way to eat chicken and tick the boxes for female hormone balance. Chicken meat is high in heme iron (the more easily absorbed iron from food). This refreshing salad contains plenty of female hormone balancing phytoestrogens and fiber.

INGREDIENTS

Polenta Chicken
- 600 g (21 oz) about 2 large organic chicken breasts
- 50 g (2 oz) coarse polenta meal (corn meal)
- 1 tablespoon dried oregano
- 1 teaspoon dried garlic granules
- 1 teaspoon dried chili flakes
- ½ teaspoon salt
- ½ teaspoon freshly ground black pepper
- 1 tablespoon extra virgin olive oil

Salad
- 400 g (14 oz) small Lebanese cucumbers, skin left on
- 2 large handfuls mint leaves, washed
- 150 g (5 oz) cooked lentils, green, black Puy or French style (cook your own or canned)
- 150 g (5 oz) fresh or frozen organic soya beans*, depodded
- 2 tablespoons lemon juice
- 3–4 tablespoons extra virgin olive oil
- 80 g (3 oz) pumpkin seeds
- 60 g (2½ oz) goat feta

*You can substitute the soya beans with fresh or frozen broad (fava) beans or peas.

1. Using a sharp knife carefully slice through the chicken breasts horizontally so you end up with 4 thin chicken breast steaks.
2. Mix the polenta meal with the oregano, dried garlic, dried chili, salt and pepper. Coat the outside of all the chicken breasts with the polenta mixture.
3. Heat a large frying pan/skillet on medium and add 1 tablespoon extra virgin olive oil.
4. Place the chicken breasts into the pan and cook for about 4 minutes. Turn the breasts over to cook for another 2 minutes. Ensure they are cooked through before taking off the heat.
5. While the chicken is cooking, cut the cucumber into really thin strips, using a mandolin or large potato peeler. Place into a large bowl.
6. Finely chop the mint leaves and add to the cucumber. Then add the lentils and beans.
7. Mix together the lemon juice and extra virgin olive oil and add to the salad gently mixing everything together.
8. Stack the salad on your serving plate and scatter the pumpkin seeds and feta over the top.
9. Slice up your chicken and add to the dish.

Cauliflower Chana Masala (V) *Serves 4*

Your body will breathe a sigh of relief when it eats this dish. It has an abundance of phytonutrients and fiber. Emma's favorite thing about this meal is that she feels nourished after she's eaten it.

INGREDIENTS

350 g (12½ oz) cooked chickpeas
500 ml (16 fl oz) chickpea cooking liquid
1 teaspoon cumin seeds
2 tablespoons extra virgin olive oil
1 red onion, finely chopped
3 cm (1 inch) knob fresh ginger, washed and roughly chopped (no need to remove skin)
2 long green chilis, split, seeds removed, if you don't like it too hot
4 large garlic cloves, peeled and crushed
1 bunch fresh coriander (cilantro)
2 heaped teaspoons ground coriander (cilantro) powder
1 heaped teaspoon ground cumin powder
1 heaped teaspoon turmeric powder
Big pinch of cardamom powder
400 g (14 oz) cherry tomatoes, washed
400 g (14 oz) fresh cauliflower, washed and cut into small florets
1 heaped teaspoon garam masala powder
1 heaped teaspoon salt
1 small lemon

Topping
Natural unsweetened yogurt
Poppadums

1. If you are cooking your own chickpeas, save 500 ml (16 fl oz) of cooking liquid for this recipe.
2. If you're using canned chickpeas, drain and put them into a saucepan with 500 ml (16 fl oz) of water. Bring to the boil and simmer for 10 minutes to soften them. Turn off the heat and save the cooking liquid.
3. Put the oil and cumin seeds into a large frying pan/skillet or saucepan, that has a lid. Turn the heat to medium and fry for about 1 minute. Add the onion, turn the heat down to low and cook for about 5 minutes until softening.
4. Wash the coriander. Roughly chop the roots and lower stems, saving the leaves to garnish.
5. In a food processor blend the ginger, garlic, chili, coriander roots, stems and some of the leaves until a rough paste forms. Add this to the pan, turn the heat to medium low and stir to softly cook.
6. After a couple of minutes add the dry spices – coriander, cumin, turmeric and cardamom powder, stirring to combine, watching that the mixture doesn't stick on the base of the pan.
7. Blend the tomatoes in the food processor (no need to rinse it) until they are broken up and pulp-like. Then add the pulp to the pan and stir, mixing well.
8. Stir in the cauliflower, chickpeas and cooking liquid, mixing well. Turn the heat to high, put the lid on and bring to the boil. Once boiling, turn down to a low simmer, and cook until the cauliflower is soft, about 10–15 minutes.
9. Towards the end of cooking, add the garam masala, salt, and lemon juice.
10. Prepare the poppadums as per the packet instructions.
11. Serve with yogurt and coriander leaves on top of each serving. Accompany with the poppadums.

Note: If you have leftovers, it is great to freeze in portions for when you want a quick meal.

Roasted Beetroot and Cauliflower Salad (V)

Serves 2

This salad is so tasty, nutritious and filling, it's ideal to eat on its own. However, Emma often pairs it with some small white fish fillets. Beetroot provides detoxification, anti-inflammatory and antioxidant support throughout our body. Beetroot and cauliflower are especially helpful to the liver, assisting with the removal of toxins.

INGREDIENTS

Salad
- 320 g (11½ oz) raw beetroot or 200 g (7 oz) cooked peeled beetroot
- ½ cauliflower – 600 g (21 oz), washed and cut into small florets
- 1 tablespoon extra virgin olive oil
- Salt and freshly ground pepper
- 30 g (1½ oz) almonds
- 1 tablespoon cumin seeds
- 2 tablespoons pumpkin seeds
- ½ bunch parsley leaves, washed

Dressing
- 1 tablespoon lemon juice
- 1 heaped tablespoon tahini
- 1 heaped tablespoon unsweetened organic yogurt

1. Set your oven to 180°C (350°F) fan forced or 200°C (400°F) regular.
2. Chop the stems off the beetroots and thoroughly wash any soil off. No need to peel them.
3. Put the beetroots on a baking tray and roast in the oven for 1 hour or until they are slightly soft to touch. This depends on what size they are. If they are baby beetroot, they will probably need about 30–40 minutes in the oven. If they are large, about 90 g (3½ oz), they will need 1 ¼ hours to cook. Under rather than overcook the beetroots to help retain their nutrients.
4. Toss the cauliflower in olive oil with a good pinch of salt and pepper. Put on a separate baking tray, lined with baking/parchment paper. Roast in the oven for 25 minutes or until it is slightly golden on the edges.
5. For the last 5 minutes of cooking time, toss the almonds, cumin and pumpkin seeds onto another tray and lightly roast in the oven.
6. Remove all trays from the oven and allow the beetroot, cauliflower, almonds and seeds to cool to room temperature.
7. In a large salad bowl, mix the lemon juice, tahini and yogurt. If the mixture is too thick, add a little water so that the dressing is the consistency of thin custard. Chop the parsley and add to the salad bowl.
8. Once the beetroot has cooled, peel off the skin and cut into large bite sized pieces.
9. Add the beetroot, cauliflower and half the almond, cumin and pumpkin seed mix to the salad bowl. Using your hands, gently mix the dressing through the vegetables.
10. Divide the salad between 2 serving plates and sprinkle with the remaining almonds and seeds. Accompany with a wedge of lemon.

We suggest serving this with 2 portions of fresh fish.

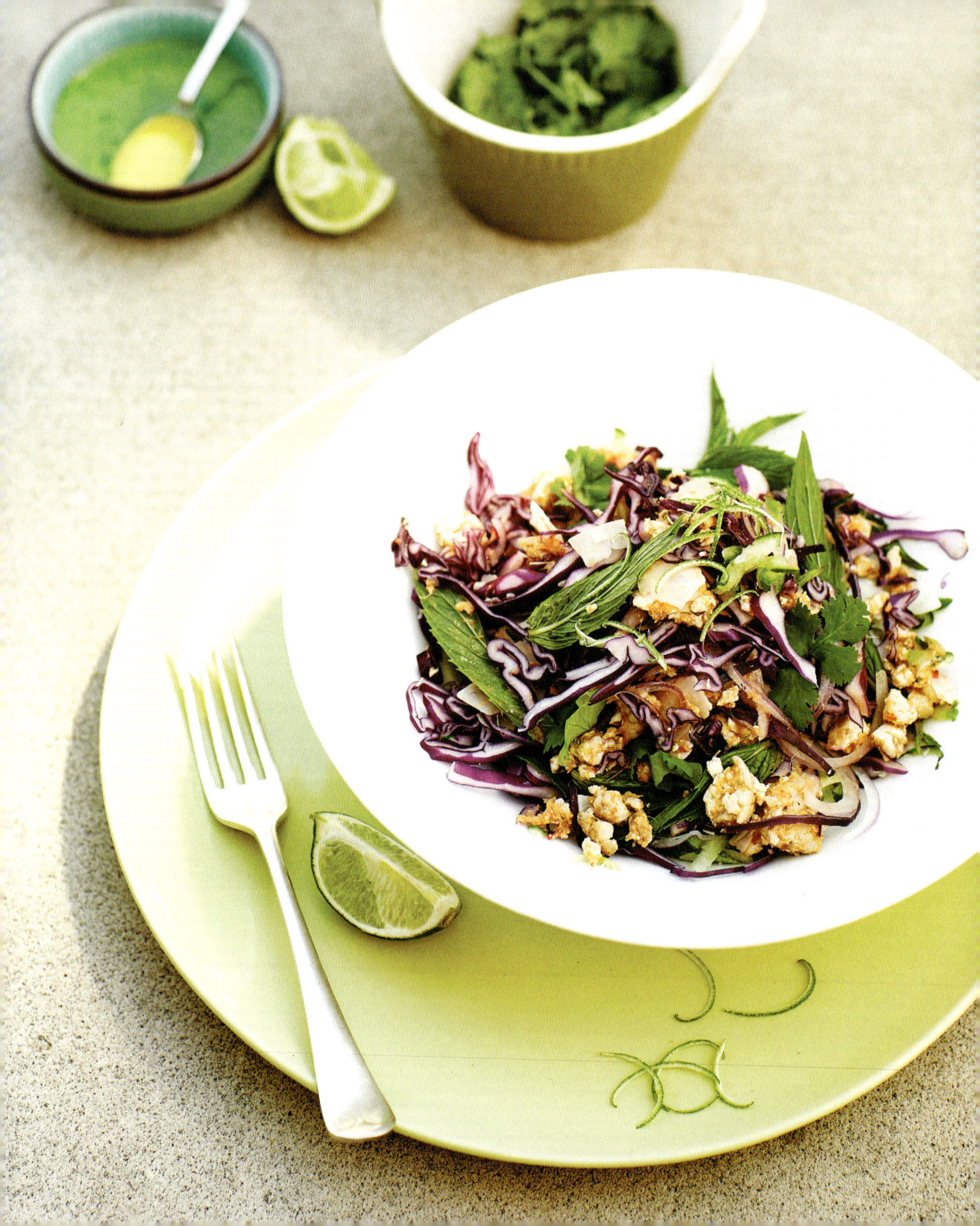

Fragrant Larb Salad
Serves 4

Larb is a minced meat Thai salad. This salad is loosely based on the traditional recipe. It's full of lovely fresh ingredients with Emma's version having even more healthful elements to benefit your body. There are a lot of ingredients in this recipe and it is easy to make. The flavor is fantastic!

INGREDIENTS
- 80 g (3 oz) spring onions
- 2 fresh kefir lime leaves with the woody center vein removed
- 1 bunch fresh coriander (cilantro) roots and stems
- 1 large long red chili, finely chopped
- 3 cm (1 inch) knob of fresh ginger, washed and coarsely grated with skin on
- 1 stem of lemongrass – 15 cm (6 inch) long
- 1 large garlic clove, peeled
- 2–3 tablespoons coconut oil
- 40 g (2 oz) crushed macadamia nuts
- 400 g (14 oz) fresh organic chicken, turkey or fish fillet mince
- 2 large fresh limes, zest and juice
- 100 g (3½ oz) organic firm tofu, crumbled
- 2 tablespoons Thai fish sauce
- 1 large handful of fresh coriander (cilantro) leaves

Salad
- 2 large handfuls fresh mint leaves
- ¼ purple cabbage, finely shredded
- ¼ red onion, peeled and very finely sliced
- 2 Lebanese cucumbers, coarsely grated with the skin on
- 30 g (1 oz) dried unsweetened coconut chips
- 1 large fresh lime, juiced
- 1 tablespoon extra virgin olive oil
- Pinch salt and freshly ground pepper

1. Prepare the salad ingredients – mint, cabbage, onion, cucumber and coconut chips. Place in a salad bowl.
2. Wash the coriander really well. Cut the roots and stems off, saving the leaves for after cooking.
3. Remove the woody outer bark from the lemongrass stalk, leaving the inner soft stem.
4. Put the coriander roots and stems, lemongrass, spring onions, kefir lime, chili, ginger and garlic in a blender and pulse until all ingredients are chopped.
5. Heat the coconut oil in a wok or large frying pan on medium heat. Add the macadamia nuts, tossing for a minute. Then add the mince, tofu, chopped mix and lime zest.
6. Stir until the mince is cooked, about 2–3 minutes.
7. Turn off the heat and add the lime juice, coriander leaves and fish sauce. Stir to combine.

To make salad
1. Mix the lime juice, olive oil, salt and pepper. Then toss through the salad ingredients. Divide the salad between your serving bowls and top with the cooked mince mixture.
2. Serve with brown rice, if you wish. Add a splash of soy sauce or tamari, if you like a more salty flavor.

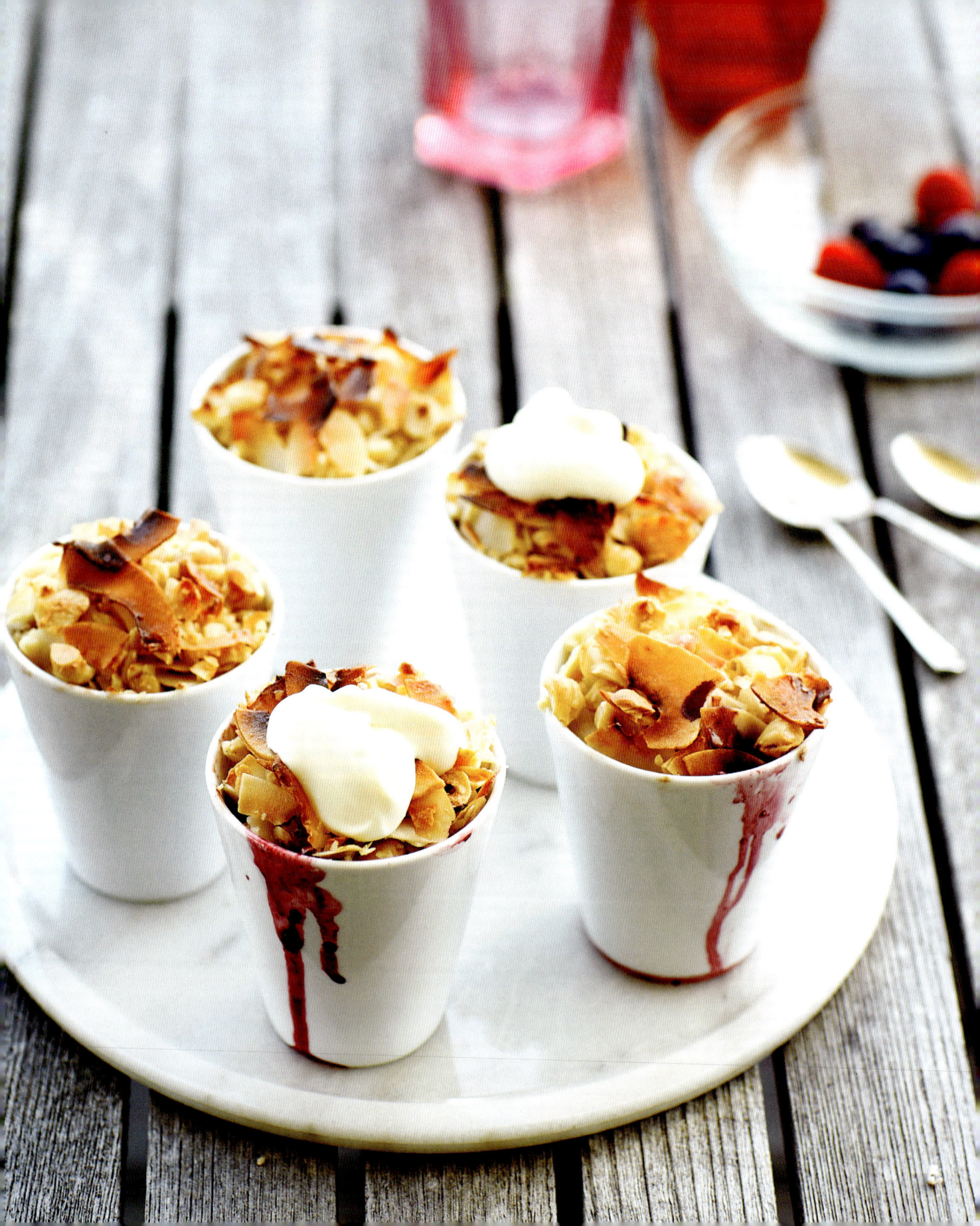

SWEET THINGS

·Zesty Lime and Ginger Balls· Makes about 15

INGREDIENTS
2 small bananas
130 g (4½ oz) cashew nuts (or other nuts of choice)
140 g (4½ oz) dried apricots (sulfur dioxide free)
Zest from 2 large limes
6 teaspoons finely grated fresh ginger
40 g (2 oz) desiccated coconut, plus extra for coating

1. Put the cashews into a food processor and grind well.
2. Add the bananas and apricots and process into a rough paste.
3. Then add the lime, ginger and desiccated coconut. Blend further.
4. Check the consistency of the paste. It needs to be firm enough to form a ball. It will still be a sticky mixture, but if too soft add in some more coconut.
5. Roll the balls and toss lightly in the extra coconut.
6. Chill in the fridge to firm before eating.

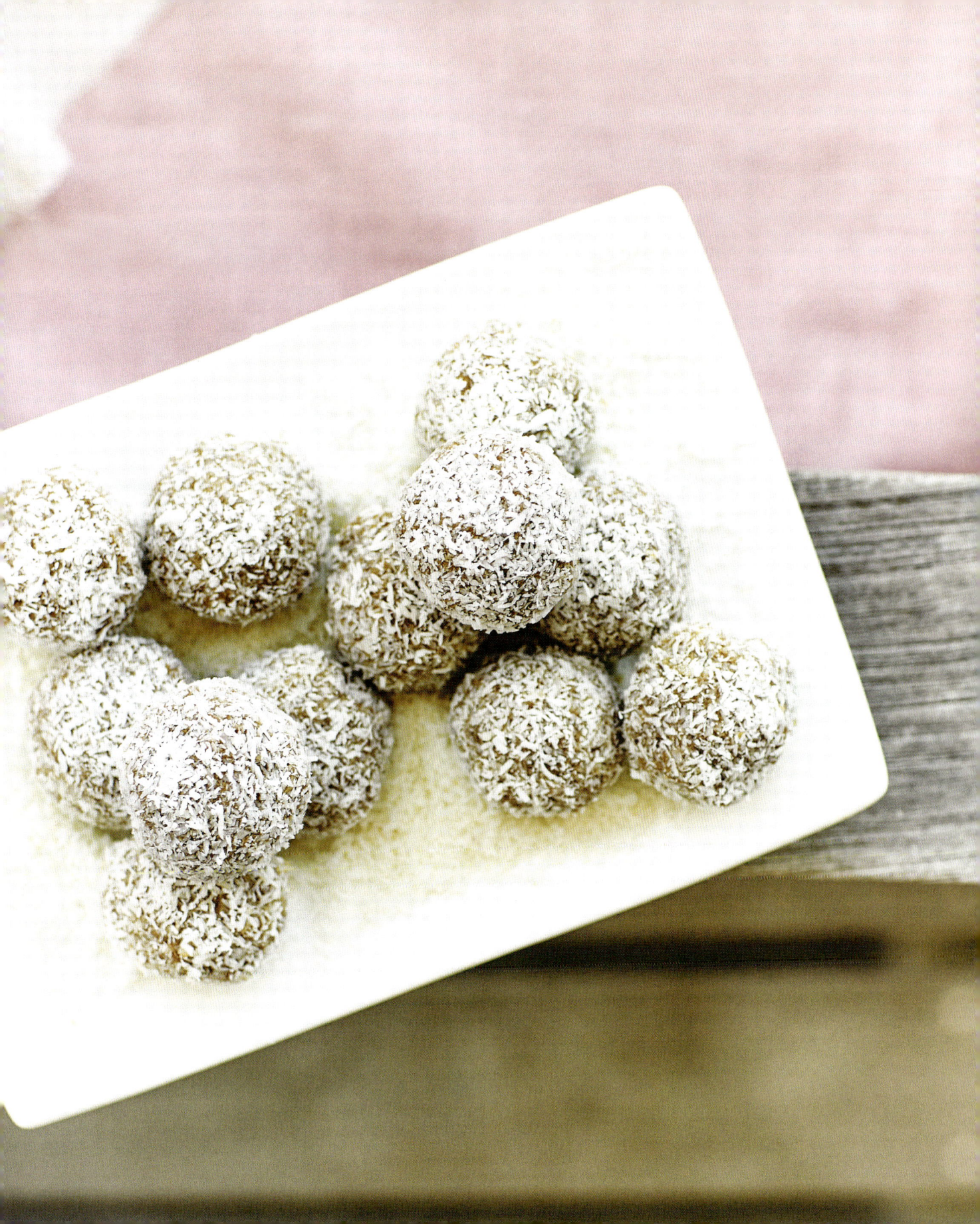

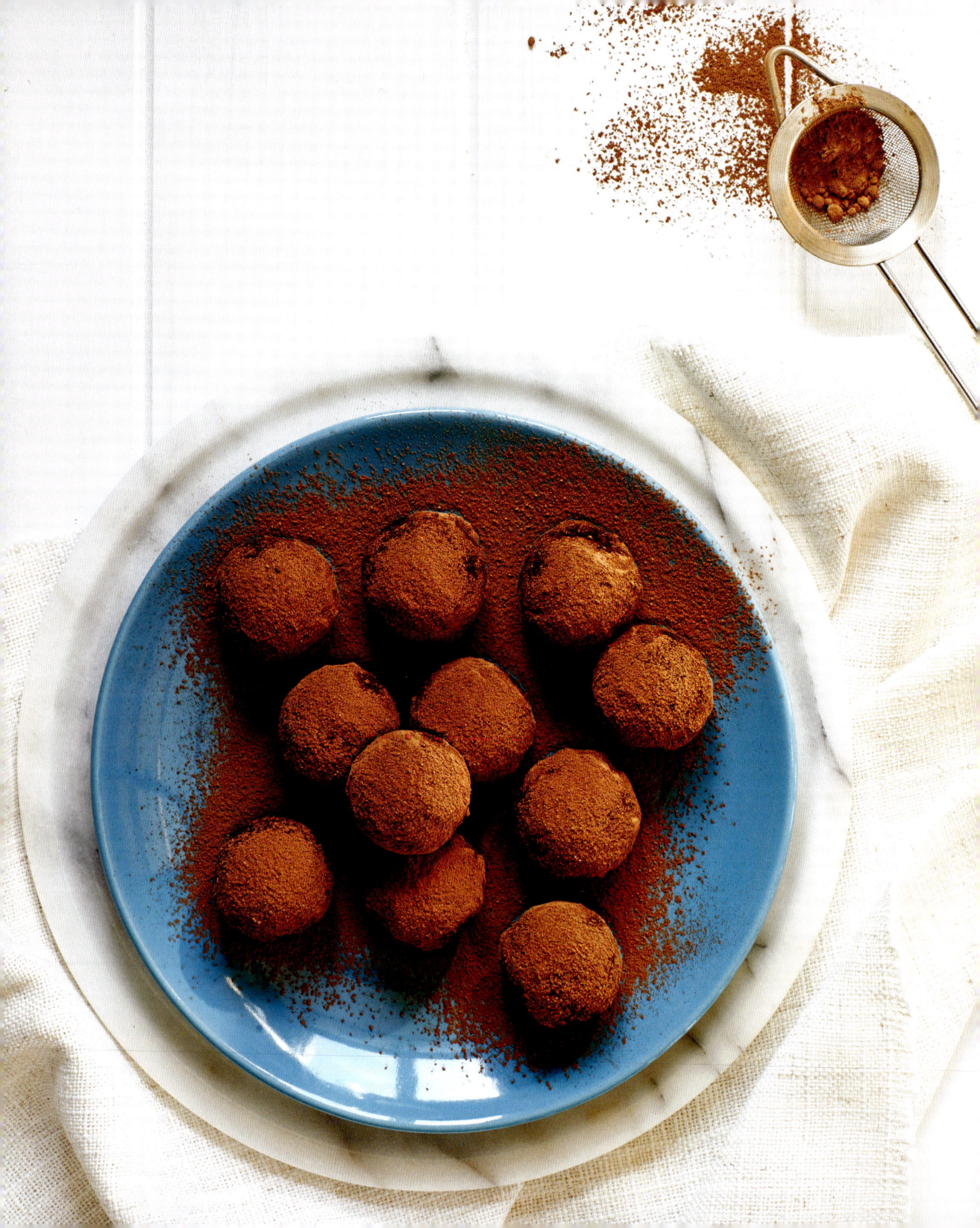

Orange and Cacao Balls
Makes about 20

The orange zest in these balls really comes through the day after you've made them. The orange flavor highlights the chocolate taste and the two go so well together. Use up the orange flesh in a salad, such as Warm Beetroot, Chickpea and Red Cabbage Salad (recipe page 97).

INGREDIENTS
4 tablespoons raw cacao or cocoa powder
200 g (7 oz) almonds
180 g (6 oz) pitted Medjool dates
2 tablespoons almond butter
2 tablespoons black chia seeds
Zest from 1 organic orange
Pinch of salt

1. Pop everything into a food processor and blend really well, until the almonds are like coarse meal.
2. Using your hands, pick up a small amount of mixture and squeeze and roll it into a ball, a little smaller than a golf ball.
3. Store these goodies in the fridge or freezer, in an airtight container.
4. Alternatively pack the mixture into a paper-lined small brownie tin (about 18 cm x 18 cm/7 inch x 7 inch) and press down firmly. Let this mixture rest in the fridge for about ½ an hour to set firm. Then use a cookie cutter to cut out shapes or cut into small squares with a knife.

•Warm Fruit Salad with Nut Crumble• Serves 6

This delicious pudding uses whatever fruit is particularly in season when you make it. Emma likes to use stone fruit in summer, and pears in winter, since neither fruit need much cooking time. You are literally warming it up and lightly toasting the top.

INGREDIENTS
250 g (9 oz) fresh peaches or pears, about 2, washed, de-stoned or cored and roughly chopped. No need to peel
250 g (9 oz) fresh or frozen berries
Zest from 1 organic lime
150 g (5 oz) hazelnuts and macadamia nuts, roughly chopped
60 g (2½ oz) unsweetened coconut chips
1 tablespoon pure maple syrup or honey

1. Set your oven to 160°C (325°F) fan-forced or 180°C (350°F) regular.
2. Toss the fruit together in a bowl and add the zest from the lime.
3. Use individual ovenproof ceramic pots, about 125 ml (4 fl oz) capacity.
4. Spoon the fruit into the pots, packing it down well as you go.
5. Mix the nuts, coconut and maple syrup together in a bowl so they become sticky. Top each of the pots with the mixture.
6. Put into the oven to crisp the top and warm the fruit, about 10 minutes. This could also be done under a grill.
7. Eat with some natural unsweetened yogurt sprinkled with cinnamon or vanilla. Alternatively serve with homemade Banana Soft Serve (recipe page 150)

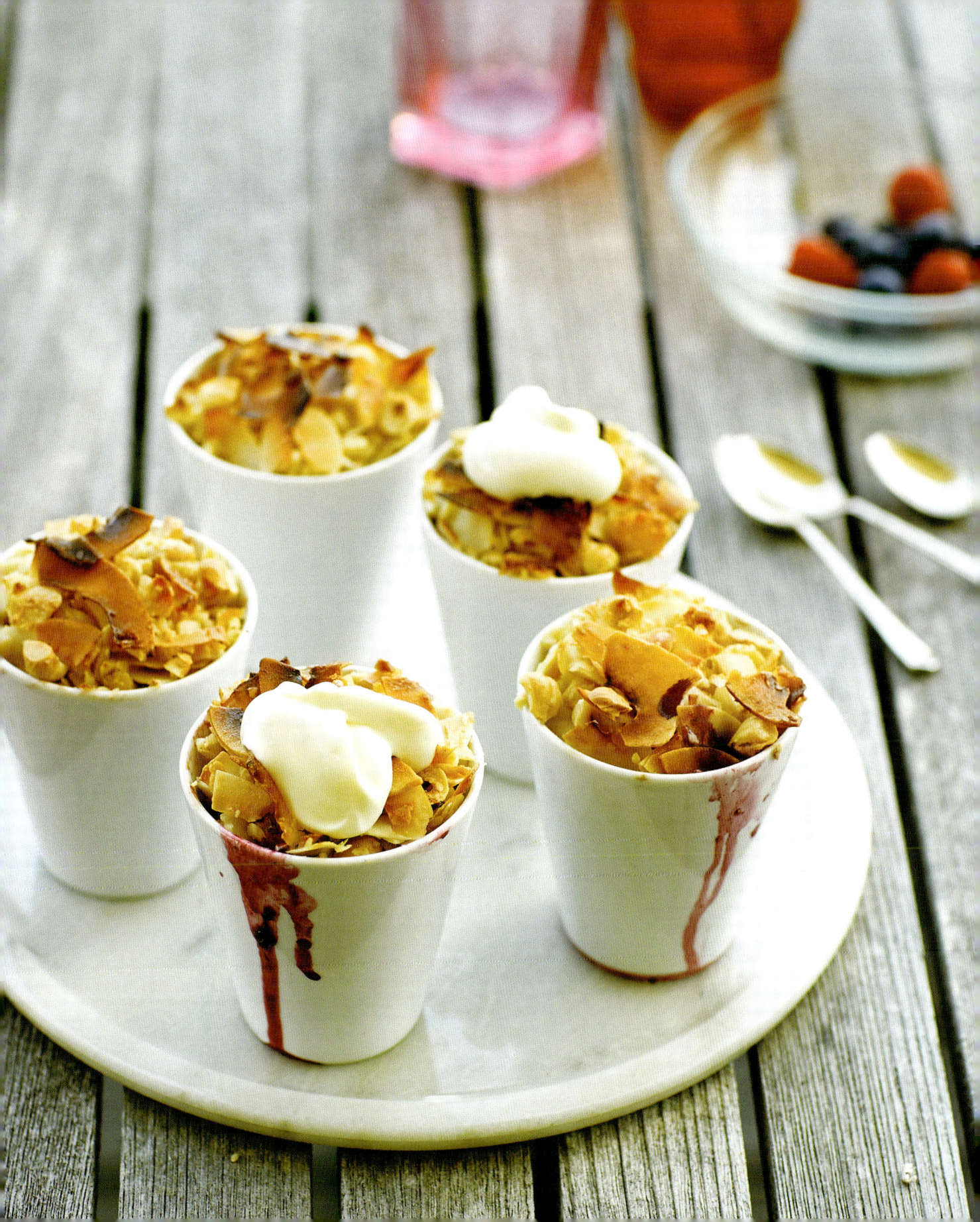

·Power-packed Banana Bites· Makes about 15

These chewy oat bites are brimming full of seeds that contain beneficial oils and minerals for female hormone balance. The oats contain fiber that helps with detoxification of toxins and excess female hormones. Just one of these bites makes a filling snack, or you could use them as a fast breakfast if you are stuck for time one morning.

INGREDIENTS
2 large ripe bananas
85 g (3 oz) organic butter
140 g (3½ oz) 100 per cent maple syrup or honey or 120 g (4½ oz) brown rice syrup
300 g (10½ oz) whole rolled oats
75 g (3 oz) pepitas
75 g (3 oz) sesame
75 g (3 oz) black chia
75 g (3 oz) sunflower seeds
Cinnamon powder for dusting

1. Set your oven at 180°C (350°F) fan forced or 200°C (400°F) regular.
2. In a mixing bowl mash the bananas.
3. Warm the butter, so it is runny. Mix with the banana and maple syrup.
4. Add the oats and seeds, mixing well. (Yes, it's lovely and messy.)
5. Take a heaped dessertspoon of the mixture and press it together firmly with your hands to form a ball. Squeeze well to make the mixture stick.
6. You will need two baking trays lined with baking/parchment paper. Place the ball on the tray and keep repeating, filling the trays.
7. Once the trays are full of the balls, use a fork to carefully press down each ball to flatten slightly. This will make the balls form a fat cookie shape. Dust the top of each bite with cinnamon powder.
8. Bake in the oven for about 20 minutes. Since all ovens can differ, watch that they don't catch and burn on the outside. You want them to be a golden color.
9. Take out of the oven and leave to go cold, as they are a bit soft whilst warm. They will remain soft and chewy in the center, with a crisp outside.
10. Once cooled, store in an airtight container. They will last several days.

·Strawberry and Coconut Cakes· Makes 10

Moist delicious cakes full of nutritious oils and phytonutrient rich berries.

INGREDIENTS

125 g (4 oz) maple syrup
2 large eggs
Zest 1 organic lemon, finely grated
90 g (3oz) almond meal/ground almonds
45 g (1½ oz) desiccated coconut
90 g (3oz) buckwheat flour
1.5 teaspoon baking powder
170 ml (6 fl oz) coconut milk
200 g (7 oz) chopped strawberries (or other berry)
2 tablespoons shredded coconut
2 tablespoons sunflower seeds
Coconut flakes and sunflower seeds, to scatter on top

1. Preheat your oven to 180°c (325°F) fan forced, 200°c (350°F) regular.
2. Put the maple syrup, eggs, lemon zest, almond meal, desiccated coconut, buckwheat flour, baking powder, and coconut milk into a food processor or mixing bowl.
3. Mix together until well combined.
4. Remove the blade from the food processor (if using), and add in the strawberries, shredded coconut and sunflower seeds. Stir to combine but try not to break up the strawberries.
5. If using a muffin tin, lightly oil up 10 regular sized muffin holes or use cake paper cases (3½ oz size)
6. Put a heaped tablespoon of mixture into each muffin whole or paper case, then scatter some flaked coconut and sunflower seeds over the top.
7. Bake for 20 minutes, then take out of the oven and allow the cakes to cool to room temperature before removing from the tin.

NOTE: Emma likes to serve these cakes with some unsweetened natural Greek-style yogurt and lots of extra berries.

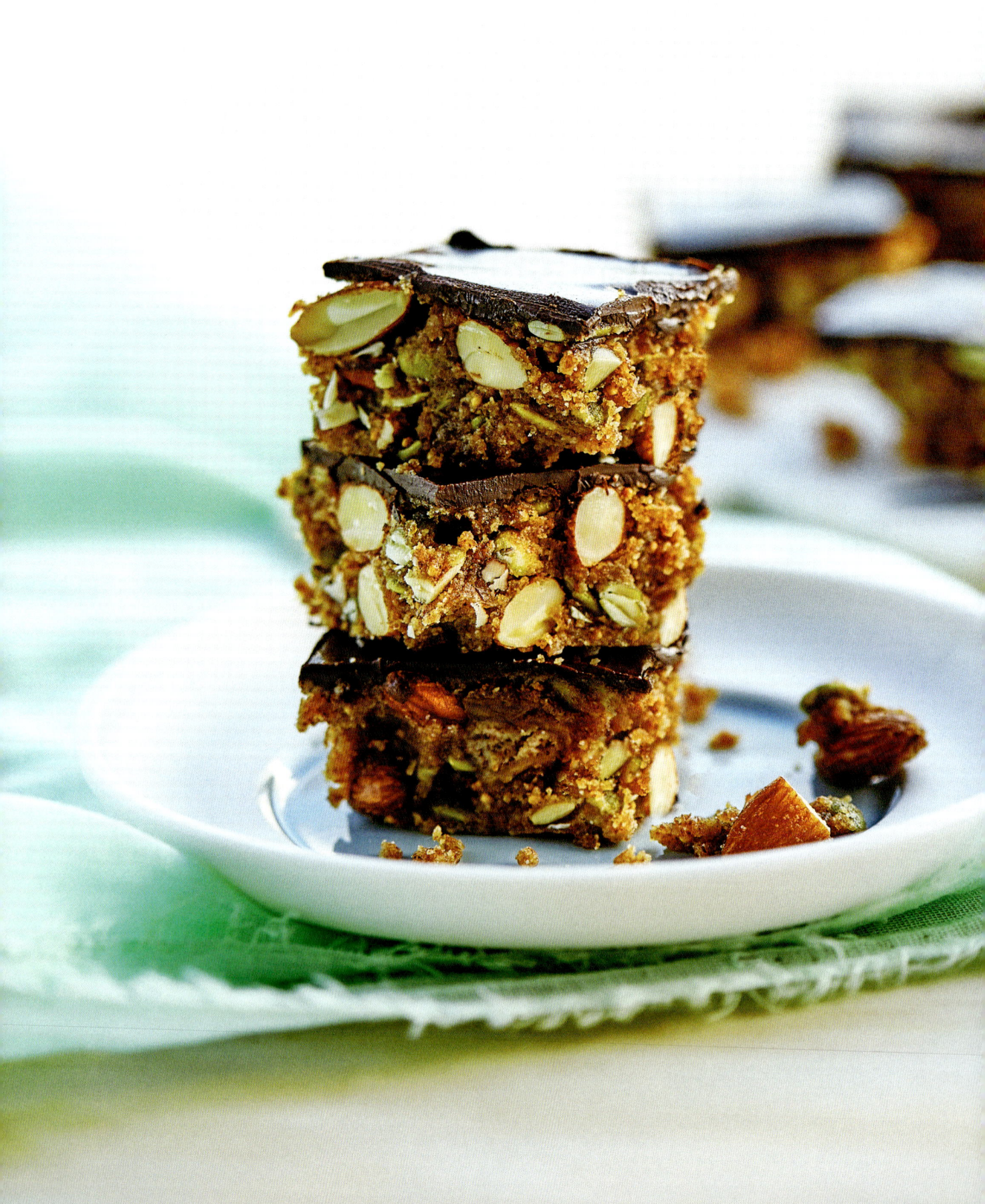

Fig and Ginger Slice

Makes about 30

This is a delicious slice cut into small bite size pieces. It is perfect to have as a snack between meals or after a meal. They are a great way to eat beneficial nuts and seeds with extra flavor. This slice freezes whole or in portions really easily.

INGREDIENTS

- 12 dried figs
- 100 g (3½ oz) 90 per cent dark chocolate
- 125 g (4½ oz) raw pumpkin seeds (pepitas)
- 150 g (5 oz) almonds
- 3 tablespoons natural coconut oil or organic butter
- 250 g (9 oz) nut butter
- 1 tablespoon fresh ginger, finely grated
- Shaved coconut

1. Soak the figs in warm water for about 10–15 minutes, then drain and finely chop.
2. Slowly melt the chocolate by putting it into a bowl placed over the top of a saucepan with about 3 cm of water gently simmering on low heat.
3. If you've got the time, lightly toast the almonds and pepita seeds in a dry frying pan on medium heat. Occasionally toss them around the pan, for about 5 minutes or roast them in an oven set at 150°C (300°F) for 15 minutes. This intensifies the lovely flavors of the nuts.
4. Into a large saucepan add the coconut oil and figs. Warm, on a low to moderate heat, for a couple of minutes mixing well. Then add the nuts and seeds, nut butter and ginger. Mix well so everything binds together.
5. Take off the heat and tip this mixture into a paper lined square tin, approximately 20 cm x 20 cm (8 inch x 8 inch).
6. Press the mixture down firmly, flattening it with the back of your hand.
7. Pour over the warmed chocolate, allowing it to thinly cover the whole top.
8. Scatter over some shaved coconut or desiccated coconut or leave bare on top.
9. Chill in the fridge for a couple of hours before cutting into bite size pieces.
10. Store in an airtight container, in the fridge, for up to 2 weeks.

•Mango and Flaxseed Soft Serve• Serves 4–6

This is a way to enjoy your ice cream and gain benefits from it at the same time!

INGREDIENTS

2 mangoes, seed removed and frozen
250 ml (8 fl oz) quality milk, e.g. homemade nut milk
2 heaped tablespoons flaxseed (linseed), ground finely
2–4 Medjool dates, pitted
½ teaspoon vanilla extract
2 heaped tablespoons natural unsweetened yogurt (goat, sheep, organic cow, buffalo or coconut)

1. In a food processor, blend the ground flaxseed, vanilla, milk, yogurt and dates until smooth and custard like. The ground flaxseed forms a custard consistency.
2. Check the taste. It should taste a bit like vanilla custard, but only faintly sweet. If not sweet enough for your taste add a tablespoon of honey or 100 per cent maple syrup. Remember, you will be adding mango, which will make it sweeter.
3. Add the frozen mango and blend well. This will make a cold soft serve consistency.
4. You can eat it straight away. In fact, it is so much better eaten freshly made. Alternatively put the mixture into a container with a lid, then into the freezer.
5. Leave in your freezer for an hour, until it has set a bit firmer. When you take it out, blend the ice crystals into the mixture to achieve a smooth soft ice cream texture and either serve or refreeze.
6. This is great on its own, with berries or with the Divine Chocolate Cake (recipe page 155).

Notes:
- If using fresh mango, prepare it the day before and freeze overnight. To prepare the mango, cut the flesh from either side of the seed, cross-cut the flesh with a knife and scoop the mango from the skin. Yields about 200 g (7 oz) per mango. Alternatively purchase frozen mango.
- To make your own Nut Milk see recipe page 29.
- You can make this with banana. Replace the mango with 2 large ripe bananas, peeled and frozen over night. I like the banana ice cream in a small bowl, drizzled with ½ teaspoon of 100 per cent pure maple syrup, and scattered with 4 crushed Brazil nuts.
- You could also try peanut butter and banana flavor by adding 2 tablespoons of quality peanut butter, rippled through the mixture before eating or freezing.
- Coconut ice cream. Alternatively use coconut milk and make coconut ice cream.
- Vanila ice cream. If you'd like a plain vanilla ice cream to use in Iced Coffee (see recipe page 158), then make the vanilla custard as per the recipe above (leaving out the mango) and freeze using an ice cream maker, if you have one. Alternatively, follow the instructions for making this soft serve and remove it from the freezer after 2 hours. Thoroughly mix through the ice crystals that have formed, and then place back in the freezer.
- If you are leaving these ice creams in the freezer for another day, they will set very firm. To serve them, take out of the freezer to soften for about half an hour before serving.

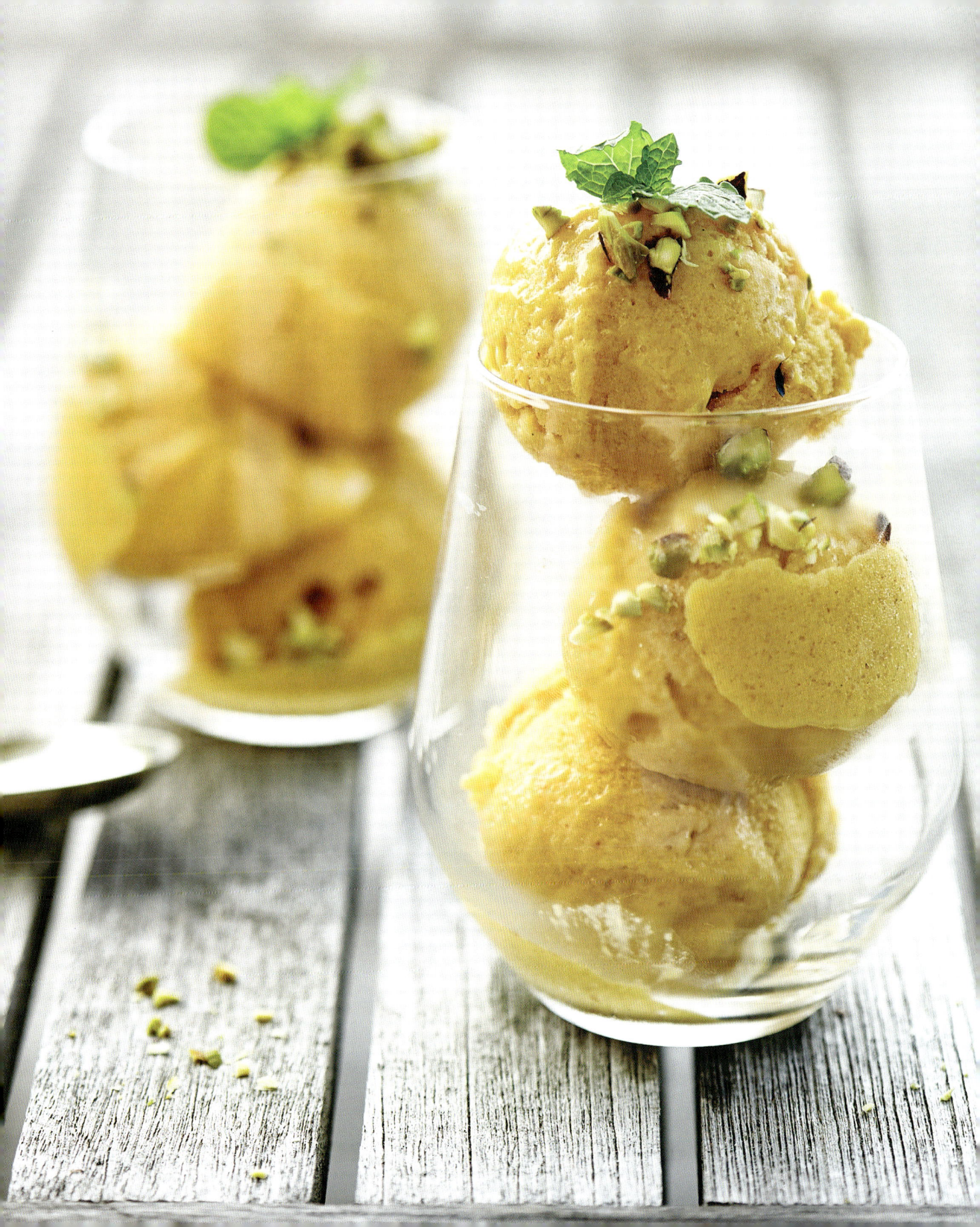

Chocolate Mousse *Serves 6*

Just try before you judge it based on its ingredients! It really does make a delicious chocolate mousse. The avocado contains boron, a trace mineral that plays a role in female hormone balance and bone health, in particular through menopause. Plus the oil in avocados has anti-inflammatory effects, and the good levels of vitamin B5 supports adrenal gland function.

INGREDIENTS

- 2 large ripe avocados
- 95 g (3 oz) honey or 100 per cent natural maple syrup or 130 g (4½ oz) brown rice syrup
- 2 tablespoons smooth macadamia or smooth almond nut butter
- 1 teaspoon vanilla extract or scraped vanilla seeds from half a pod
- 35 g (1½ oz) cacao or cocoa powder
- A pinch of salt

1. Using a spoon scrape all the avocado flesh away from the skin.
2. Pop everything into a food processor and blend until smooth and well mixed.
3. Scrape down the sides of the bowl and re-blend to make sure everything is well mixed, smooth and creamy.
4. Play around with the amount of sweetness and chocolatey-ness, if you wish, as everyone's tastes differ.
5. This mousse will not set any stiffer, so you can eat it straight away or store covered, in the fridge. It will last for 2–3 days. It is also delicious frozen and eaten as ice blocks.
6. Enjoy it with Divine Chocolate Cake (recipe page 155), Mango and Flaxseed Soft Serve (recipe page 150) or your choice of fresh berries with natural yogurt sweetened with honey or maple syrup.

Chocolate Truffles – A Very Chocolatey Hit

Makes about 15

What better way to get a chocolate fix and it's good for you.

Chocolate cravings are reported to be the most common food craving in women. Those cravings occur with hormonal changes around the time of menstruation. Cacao contains flavonoids, which have an antioxidant, as well as an anti-inflammatory, affect in the body. Cacao has a range of positive psychological effects, including enhanced cognitive function and stimulation of feelings of wellbeing and euphoria. No wonder we girls love it so much!

INGREDIENTS

- 125 g (4½ oz) ground almonds
- 50–70 g (2–3 oz) cacao or cocoa powder, plus additional for dusting
- 250 g (9 oz) pitted fresh Medjool dates or pitted dried dates
- 3–4 tablespoons coconut oil, warmed
- ½ teaspoon salt
- ½ teaspoon vanilla extract or scraped vanilla seeds from a pod

1. Put all ingredients into a food processor and mix thoroughly.
2. If the mixture is a bit crumbly, add another tablespoon of coconut oil or warm water. The water makes the mixture a bit sticky.
3. Take a dessertspoon of the mixture, a little smaller than a golf ball, and press firmly together in your hands to form a ball. Roll to smooth off.
4. Keep repeating until all the mixture is used. Put them in the fridge to set. Once set, dust with cocoa powder.
5. These can be very chocolatey. If not to your taste, reduce the amount of cocoa or cacao powder.

Note: If using dried dates, soak them in hot water for 15 minutes, then drain. Also, if you are sensitive to caffeine, then avoid these in the evening since they contain plenty of caffeine from the cocoa.

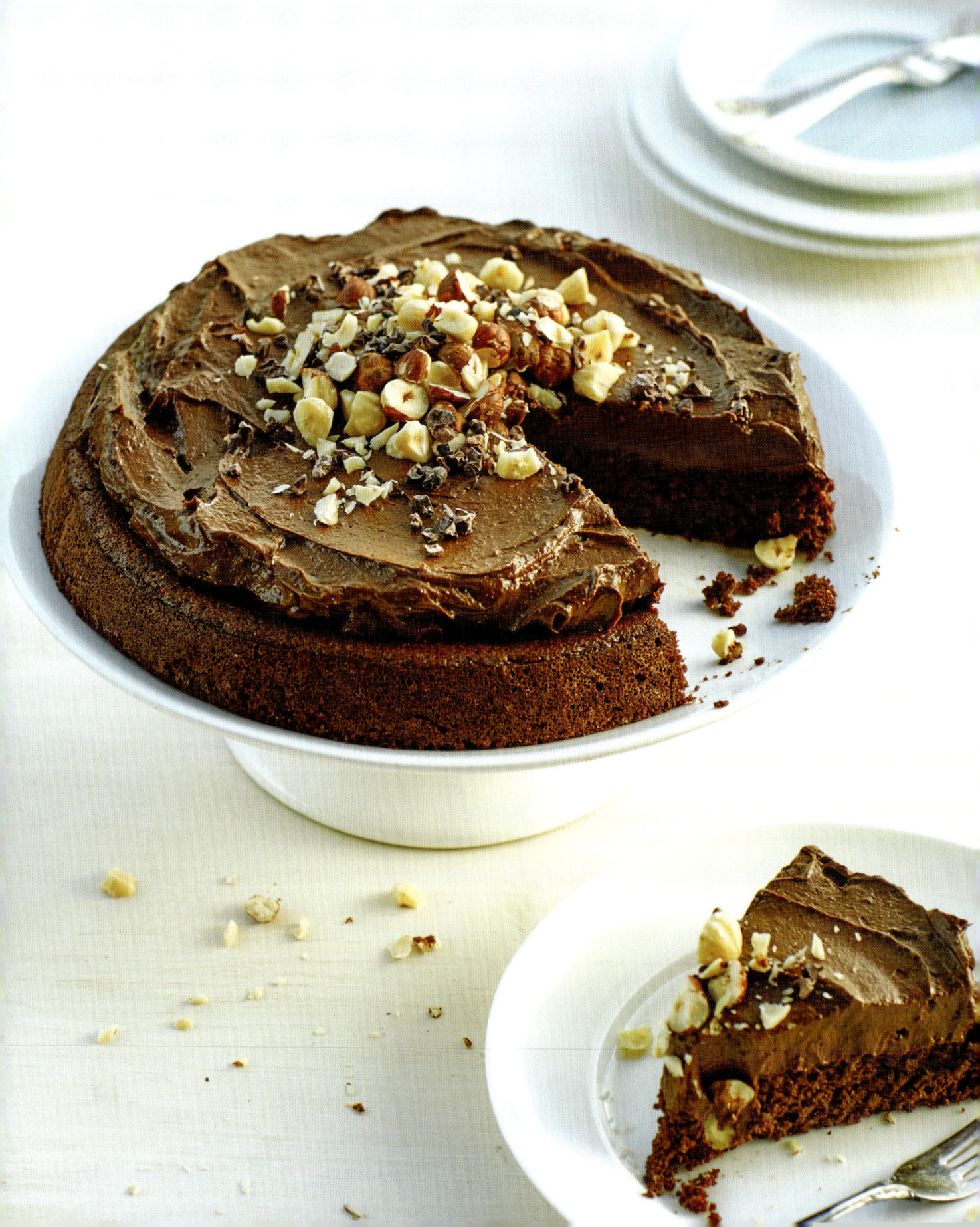

Divine Chocolate Cake • Serves 10

Not your average everyday gluten-free chocolate cake. This is one to save up for when the girls come round or you have a family gathering, We hope you and your friends enjoy it.

INGREDIENTS

- 40 g (2 oz) cacao or 60 g (2 ½ oz) cocoa powder
- 140 ml (3½ fl oz) extra virgin olive oil, plus some for the cake tin
- 50 g (2 oz) unbleached castor sugar or 60 g (2½ oz) coconut sugar
- 1 teaspoon vanilla extract or scraped seeds from half a vanilla pod
- 125 ml (4 fl oz) boiling water
- 150 g (5 oz) finely ground hazelnuts or finely ground almonds
- 1 teaspoon baking powder (aluminum-free)
- 1 pinch salt (helps to bring out the chocolate flavor)
- 3 large eggs

1. Preheat your oven to 160°C (325°F) fan forced or 180°C (350°F) regular.
2. Grease a 20 cm (8 inch) round cake tin with a little oil and line the base and sides with baking/parchment paper. You can use a small brownie tin.
3. In a bowl add the cacao, vanilla and sugar, whisking in the boiling water until you have a smooth paste. Set aside to cool a little.
4. Then add the ground nuts, the baking powder and pinch of salt. Don't bother to mix these just yet.
5. In a separate bowl, whisk the egg whites until soft peaks form.
6. Add the olive oil and egg yolks to the cacao and nut mixture. Mix together thoroughly. Then gently fold in the whisked egg whites until only just combined, trying to keep as many air bubbles as possible.
7. Pour all the cake mixture into the prepared tin, scraping down the sides of the bowl.
8. Bake for 25 minutes or until the sides are set. A cake tester should come up with a little soft cake mixture on it. Take care not to over bake this cake. Under cooked is better than over cooked.
9. Let it cool for 15 minutes out of the oven, still in its tin.
10. Consider topping with Chocolate Mousse (recipe page 152).
11. Serve with mashed berries or mango slices and coconut cream or thick natural unsweetened greek-style organic yogurt. Mango and Flaxseed Soft Serve (recipe page 150) is delicious with this.

Note: An alternative quick method is to put all the ingredients into a food processor and mix until combined. Pour into the lined cake tin and bake as per the recipe. The cake will not be as high as the previous method, but it's still great.

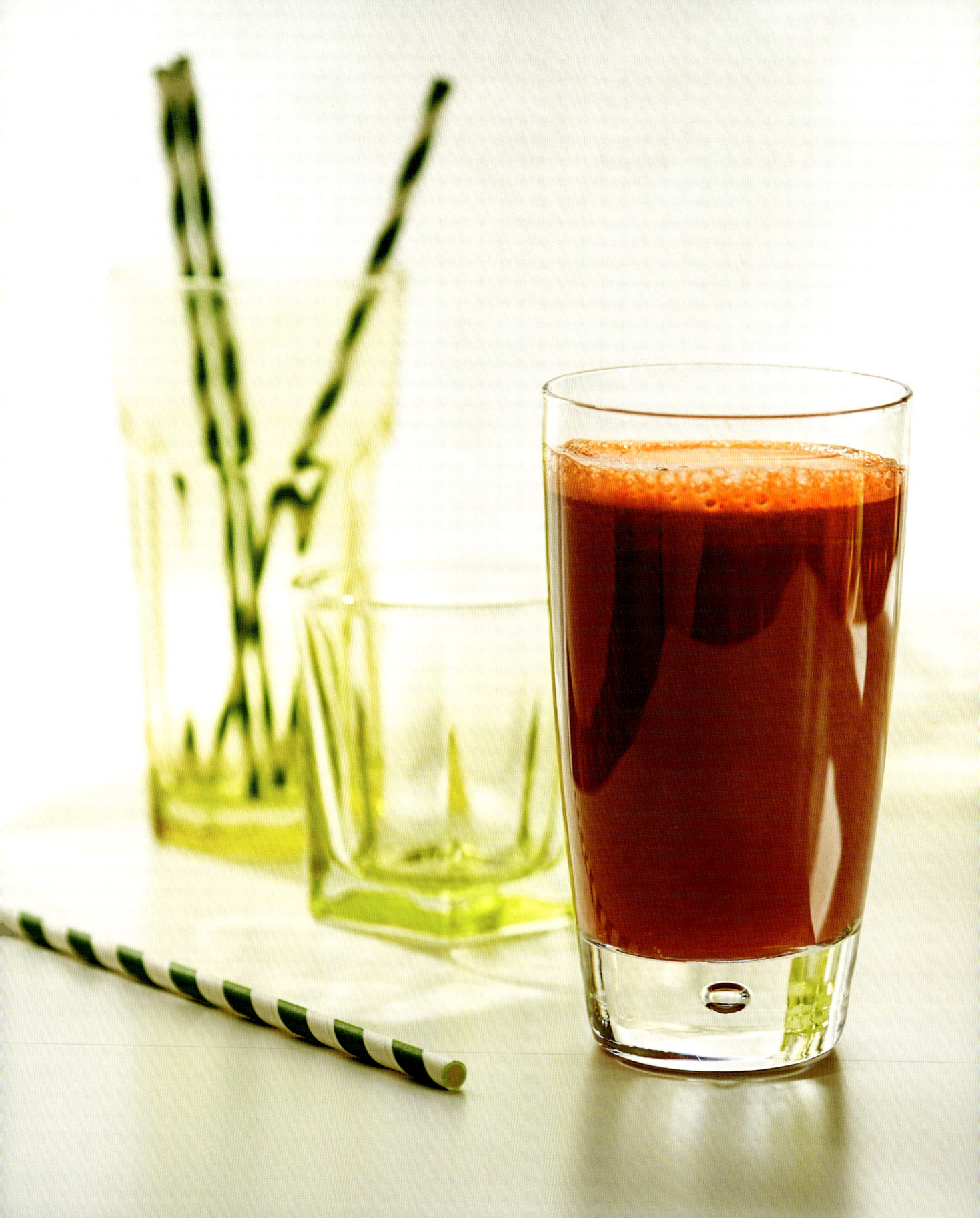

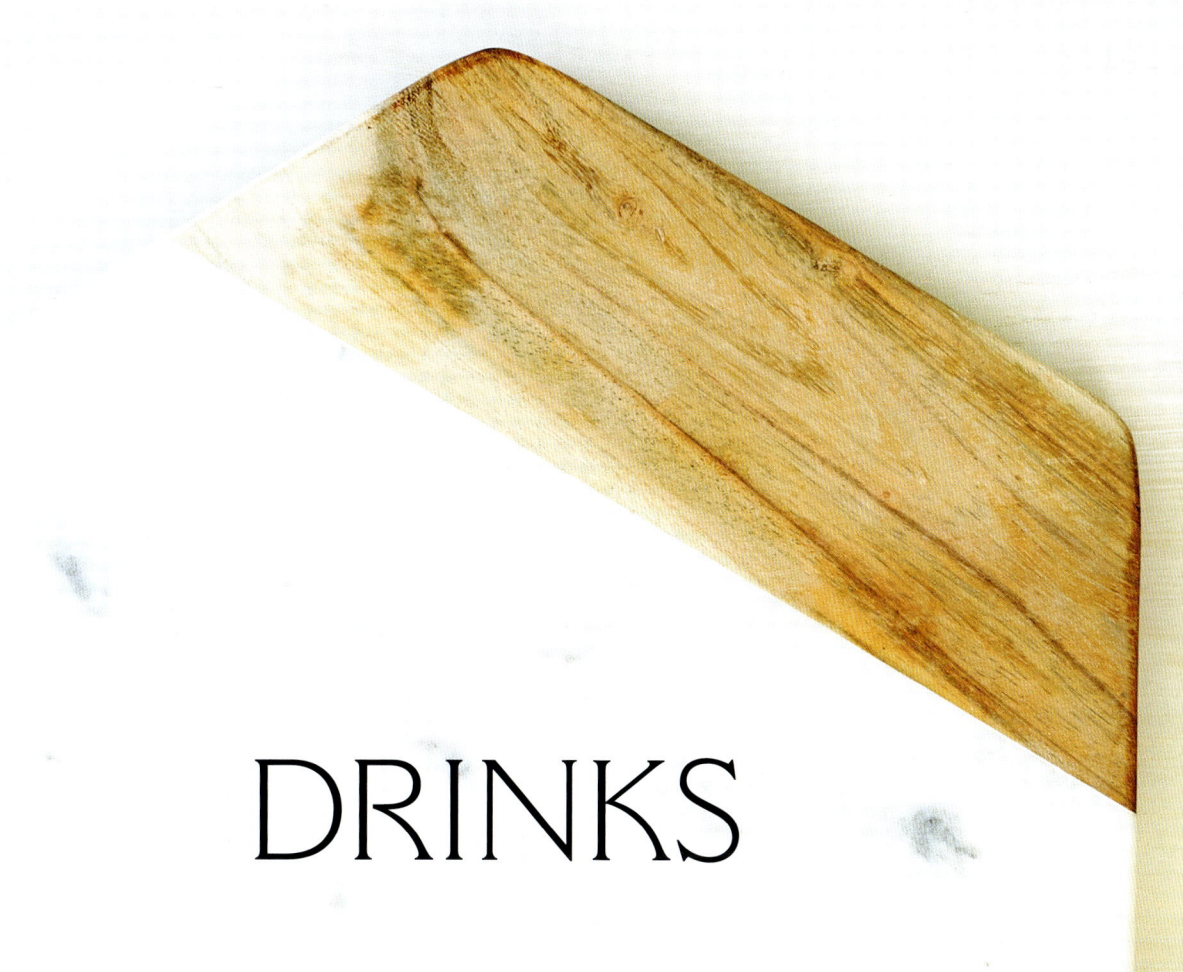

DRINKS

DRINKS

Drinks can encompass a lot of things from fresh, clean, safe drinking water to juices, milks, smoothies, soft drinks (sodas), coffee, teas, alcohol and fermented drinks such as kefir and kombucha. Some are beneficial, others not so.

Water

One of the best drinks is water. Drinking it at regular intervals during the day is important for good health. If you are blessed to live in a country that has safe drinking water, then there are plenty of ways to drink it and stay hydrated. Hydration is important for your whole body's optimal health.

Being dehydrated, even before you may realize it, means you are likely to feel tired and lack concentration. If you're not sure how much water to drink, then here's an easy calculation for your daily water needs: 30 ml per 1kg of your body weight. (This may need to be adjusted depending on your medical condition, climate and/or exercise program). This calculation is based on water and/or herbal teas, not other liquids you consume, which could include caffeinated, sugary or alcoholic drinks.

These are some of our favorite ways to spritz up water. We like to filter the water from our tap.

Mix a large glass of sparkling or still water with 2 teaspoons of organic apple cider vinegar.

Filter some water into a large glass jug or water bottle and add one of these combinations, a handful of:
- » Fresh crushed mint and strawberries
- » Fresh crushed basil and cut watermelon
- » Fresh cut limes, lemons or oranges
- » Fresh strips of cucumber

Coffee and Caffeine

There are many views about coffee – it's bad for you and it's good for you! Coffee in moderation, ideally no more than one espresso a day, can be good for you.

Research seems to indicate that coffee may help with a number of diseases, including reducing the incidence of fatty liver disease. This is based on a specific amount of coffee consumed, and doesn't address people who find they have a negative effect from consuming coffee. It is very individual.

Caffeine can increase premenstrual and menopausal symptoms. Some find it doesn't disturb their sleep, others find if they drink coffee after midday, they have disturbed sleep. While others find they 'need' coffee 'to wake them up' in the morning, but find they are then anxious and stressed during the day. Some can get migraines after consuming caffeine drinks. Others can feel more restless, while for others it relieves their headaches.

Is the coffee exacerbating over worked adrenal glands? Is it contributing to your stress, elevating cortisol and causing poor nutrient absorption in the gut?

If you think it is negatively affecting you, then try gradually going off coffee and stopping for about 4 weeks. Then reintroduce it in moderation.

Consider buying organic fair trade coffee beans because coffee is a heavily sprayed crop. It also has a reputation of poorly paying workers in some countries.

If you like the flavor, but don't like the effects of caffeine, then organic water-filtered decaffeinated coffee is also good to drink in moderation. However, even this can have an effect on hormone balance, so don't over consume it.

Consider what you are adding to your coffee in the way of milk and sweetners. Most skim milks already have added carbohydrate sugars in the form of skim milk powder to make them palatable. Review what you are consuming, and assess its nutrient value for your body's health and balance.

Here's a great way to have your occasional coffee. We love an iced coffee, especially in summer. You may enjoy this one.

·Iced Coffee· Serves 1

INGREDIENTS
1 shot of espresso coffee or 1 short black, about 40–60 ml (1–2 fl oz)
250 ml (8 fl oz) chilled Nut Milk (recipe page 29)
1 scoop homemade Flaxseed Vanilla Ice Cream (recipe page 150)
1 cup ice

1. In a tall glass add the ice and pour over the coffee.
2. Carefully add the milk, creating a swirl-like effect with it.
3. Add a scoop of homemade flaxseed vanilla icecream, and enjoy!

Teas

There is a wide range of teas to be enjoyed – black, green, matcha, white, oolong, yerba mate and herbal teas, some of which have medicinal properties.

Whilst black, green, matcha, white and oolong teas come from the same plant, there is a difference in the fermentation process. Green tea and matcha are not fermented. All contain caffeine, so, if you are caffeine sensitive you may find these teas overstimulate you causing insomnia, anxiety and irritability. Again drink them in moderation.

All these teas have some health benefits. Green tea and matcha are two of the most beneficial. Research has found the phytonutrients in green tea have many health promoting properties including boosting cardiovascular health, reducing the risk of cancer, assisting to lower cholesterol and enhancing weight loss.

Herbal teas can assist to reduce your caffeine intake. There is a wide range of herbal teas to enjoy – bergamot, chamomile, fennel, ginger, lemon myrtle, peppermint, lemongrass, rooibos and spearmint, among others. Each has a benefit.

Organic herbal teas, made warm or as iced tea, can be very refreshing.

•Ginger and Mint Iced Tea• Serves 2

INGREDIENTS
2 heaped teaspoons coarsely grated fresh ginger or dried ginger
1 handful washed fresh mint leaves or 2 teaspoons dried mint tea
A few fresh mint leaves for the iced tea glasses
500 ml (17 fl oz) water
2 cups ice

1. Heat the water to just below boiling, and then combine with the ginger and mint.
2. Leave to brew until the water is cooled.
3. Divide the ice between two tall glasses, lightly crush a few mint leaves, and add them to the glasses.
4. Strain the cooled tea over the ice, and enjoy this refreshing stimulating drink.

Medicinal Herbal Teas

There are also 'medicinal' herbal teas, which have health benefits. Here are some you may care to consider and try.
- » Adaptogens such as Withania (Ashwagandha), Siberian/Korean ginseng, licorice root and rehmannia for adrenal support
- » Dandelion root for a bitter stimulating taste and liver support
- » Dong Quai, peony, ginger and cinnamon for painful periods

- » Peppermint/spearmint or ginger, fennel seeds and chamomile blend for gut soothing and digestion
- » Black cohosh root for hot flashes
- » Sage for night sweats
- » Lavender or lemon balm, passionflower, valerian, chamomile and hops for improved sleep
- » Shatavari for increasing libido
- » Raspberry leaf for stomach cramps and painful periods
- » Bupleurum, peony, Dong Quai, and dandelion leaf for premenstrual syndrome, breast tenderness, and fluid retention
- » Schisandra berry for anti-aging effects
- » Burdock, cleavers and nettle leaf for skin and cleansing
- » Chaste tree (Vitex agnus-castus) for premenstrual syndrome, associated acne and hormone modulation
- » Skullcap, St John's Wort and vervain for nervous fatigue, emotional stress and irritability

These herbal teas can usually be found in most large health food stores or online from a trusted organic source.

Note: If you are on any medication, are pregnant or have a medical condition, we recommend you check first with your medical professional to ensure these won't cause interference.

Fermented Drinks

Fermented drinks, such as kefir and kombutcha, offer a great way to provide your body with probiotics.
Try making your own by sourcing a seller of the starter cultures.
Kefir drinks can be made from milks, water or coconut water, and can sometimes taste slightly sour or yogurt-like, if made with milk.
Kombutcha drinks can be made from teas and sugar or other sweetners. The sugar is partially fermented. They can taste subtly sharp.
When buying either drink, check they contain live bacteria, and are low in sugar (approximately less than 5 g (0.17 oz) per 100 ml (3.4 fl oz)).

Not so favourable drinks

One of the least beneficial drinks for female hormone balance is alcohol, which can increase oestrogen levels, put extra pressure on your liver's function and hamper absorption of nutrients from your gastro-intestinal tract.
The other least favourable types of drinks are soft drinks or sodas and other sugary drinks, such as cordials and commercial juices. These can disturb hormone balance, your liver's work and your mood.
We recommend you drink alcohol in moderation and avoid sugar drinks.
Here are some other favorite drinks.

•Cleansing Juice• Serves 1

This juice is for those occasions when you feel like a 'pick-me-up' juice. Your gut may feel sluggish or you may feel you want to boost your nutrient in take. This is for those times. Use up the pulp as well, in an omelette or add to the Green Egg Pies (recipe page 63).

INGREDIENTS
1 carrot
¼ beetroot
1 large celery stick
1 cm (¼ inch) ginger

1. Wash and leave the skin on the vegetables, then put them through your juice machine.
2. Make sure you drink it straight away to get the nutrients in this juice. Again you can pour this juice over ice.

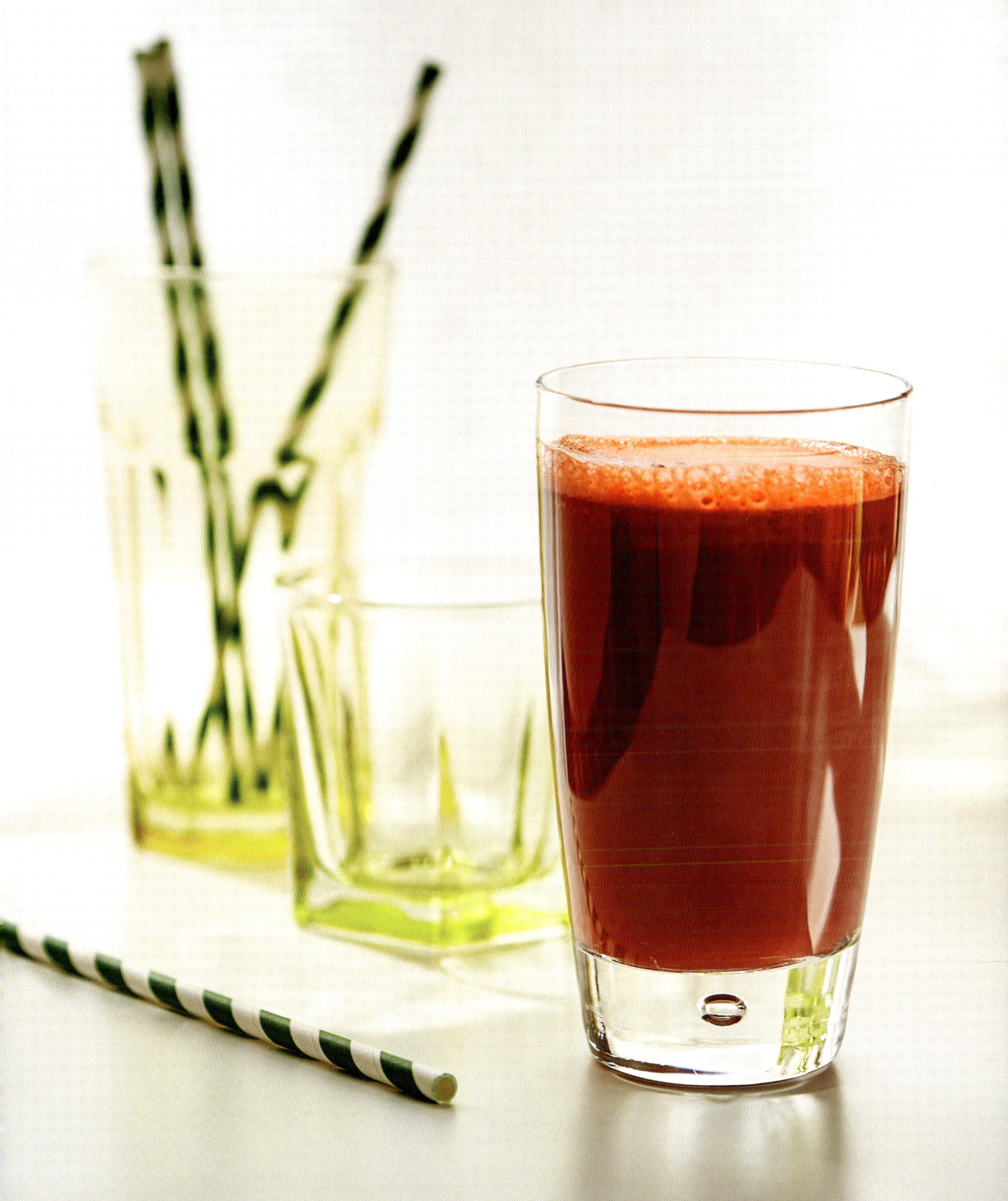

Summer Berry Smoothie *Serves 1*

This is a great berry smoothie to have as a snack, especially when berries are in season. If you want your smoothie particularly thick then use frozen berries. The flaxseed (linseed) provides a rich source of dietary fiber, good oils, lignans and isoflavones. The isoflavones provide soothing soluble dietary fiber, anti-inflammatory essential fatty acids, modulating oestrogen and help to reduce oestrogen reabsorption from the bowel.

INGREDIENTS

- 100 g (3½ oz) fresh or frozen berries (your choice of strawberries, blackberries, raspberries, black currants, mulberries)
- 250 ml (8 fl oz) nut milk or coconut water
- 1 tablespoon flaxseeds (linseeds)
- 1 teaspoon vanilla extract, or vanilla seeds scraped from ¼ of a pod
- 2 pitted Medjool dates or 2 teaspoons honey or 100 per cent pure maple syrup or organic brown rice syrup

1. Put everything into your blender and mix until the ingredients are smooth and thick.

Thick Chocolate and Chia Smoothie

Serves 2

This nourishing drink contains beneficial fats, fiber and phytonutrients in the avocado, berries, cacao and chia seeds. Together these make up a nutritious female hormone balance drink, which nourishes your ovaries and helps your body's detoxification process.

This is a snack for when you're particularly hungry or it can be made for breakfast. You can also make this smoothie into icypoles in summer.

INGREDIENTS

- 1 tablespoon organic raw cacao powder or cocoa powder
- 1 tablespoon black chia seeds
- 1 tablespoon ripe avocado flesh
- 85 g (3½ oz) frozen blueberries
- ½ fresh or frozen ripe banana
- 300 ml (10 fl oz) milk of your choice. Ideal with Nut Milk (recipe page 29)

1. Put all the ingredients into a blender and blend well.
2. The longer you leave this smoothie before drinking it, the thicker it will become. The chia seeds will swell. If it is too thick, add a little more liquid.

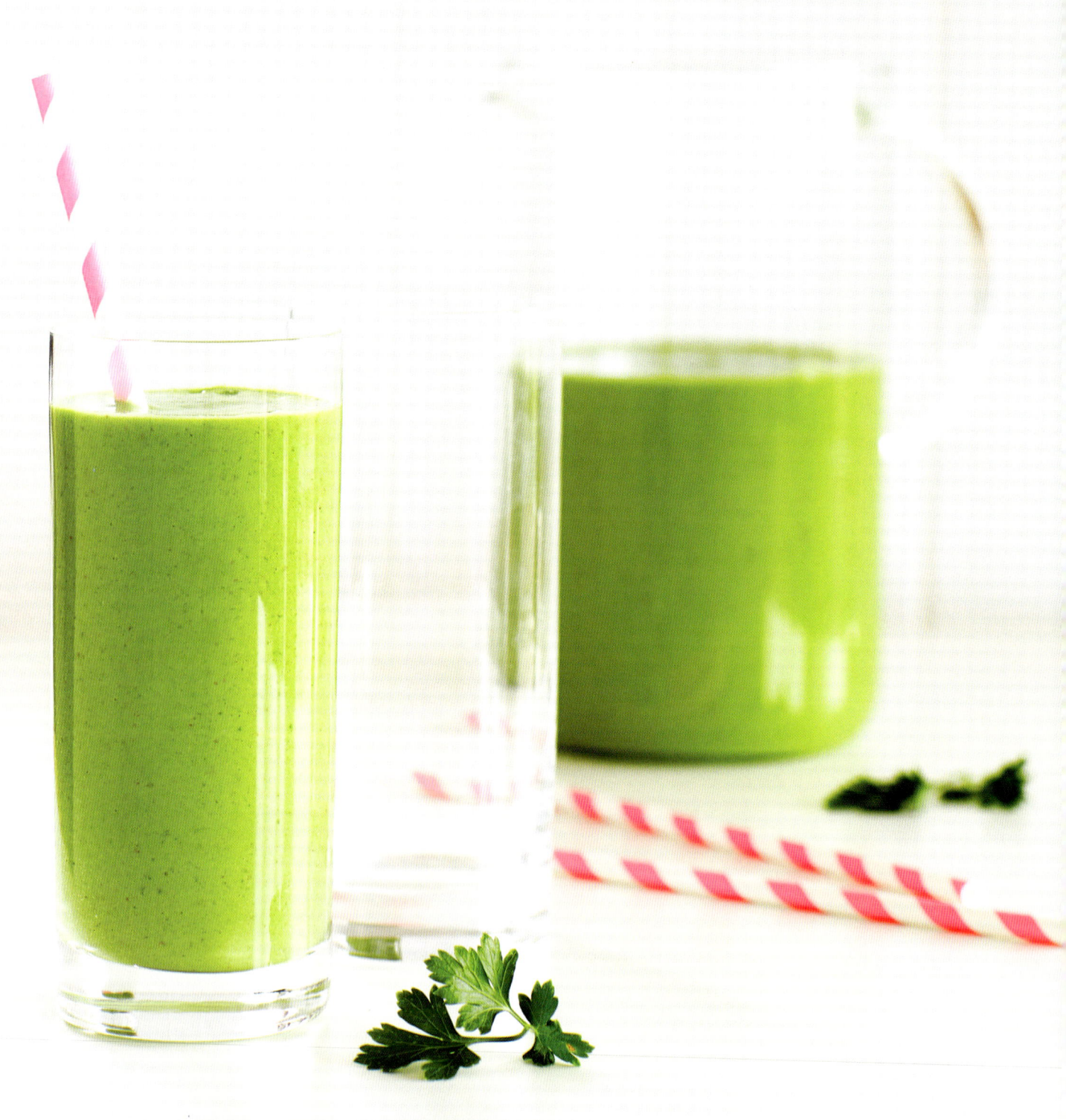

Super Green Smoothie *Serves 1*

Smoothies can be a convenient fast way to have breakfast and, if you pack in the nutrients, as these do, to heal your body's menstrual or menopausal problems, then they can be therapeutically beneficial. This smoothie contains phytonutrient rich vegetables, good oils, probiotics and prebiotics.

INGREDIENTS
1 handful spinach, kale, silverbeet or chard
¼ large ripe avocado
½ handful parsley leaves, washed
2 pitted dates
250 ml (8 fl oz) iced water
1 tablespoon flaxseeds
2 tablespoons natural unsweetened yogurt

1. In a smoothie maker or blender, blend all the ingredients together, until you get the consistency you want. Add a little ice if you wish. Drink straight away.

·Creamy Hot Chocolate· Serves 1

Cacao is the unroasted form of cocoa, which means it has a similar flavor, but is higher in the beneficial phytonutrient flavonoids and polyphenols. Cocoa still has these, but in lesser amounts.

For more about the health benefits of cacao, (see Chocolate Truffles recipe page 153).

Cacao and cocoa can be a crop that is heavily sprayed with pesticides and its workers poorly paid. So consider buying organic fair trade cacao.

A drink that we love is a homemade nut milk hot chocolate. It is especially good with cashew nut milk which is deliciously creamy.

INGREDIENTS
1 large mug of creamy nut milk
2 heaped teaspoons organic cacao powder
1–2 teaspoons raw honey, 100 per cent natural maple syrup or organic brown rice syrup

1. Warm the nut milk, but don't over heat it because it could separate and become clumpy.
2. Add the cacao and sweetner and using a small whisk, froth the hot chocolate so it is smooth, well mixed and creamy.

·Iced Turmeric Milk· Serves 1

Pepper contains the phytonutrient Piperine. This, along with the oil in the nut butter, helps the curcumin, the beneficial anti-inflamatory phytonutrient in turmeric, to be absorbed better.

We really enjoy making and drinking this with our nut milk.

INGREDIENTS
- 1 teaspoon smooth nut butter (not peanut butter, as the flavor is too strong) or 1 teaspoon of coconut oil
- 1 teaspoon turmeric powder
- 250 ml (8 fl oz) of your favorite Nut Milk (see recipe page 29)
- Pinch freshly ground black pepper
- 1 teaspoon honey or pure maple syrup or 1–2 teaspoons organic brown rice syrup

1. Mix the nut butter or oil and turmeric together. Put it into your smoothie maker along with the nut milk, pepper and honey. Blend really well, so it is frothy. Pour over ice in a tall glass.

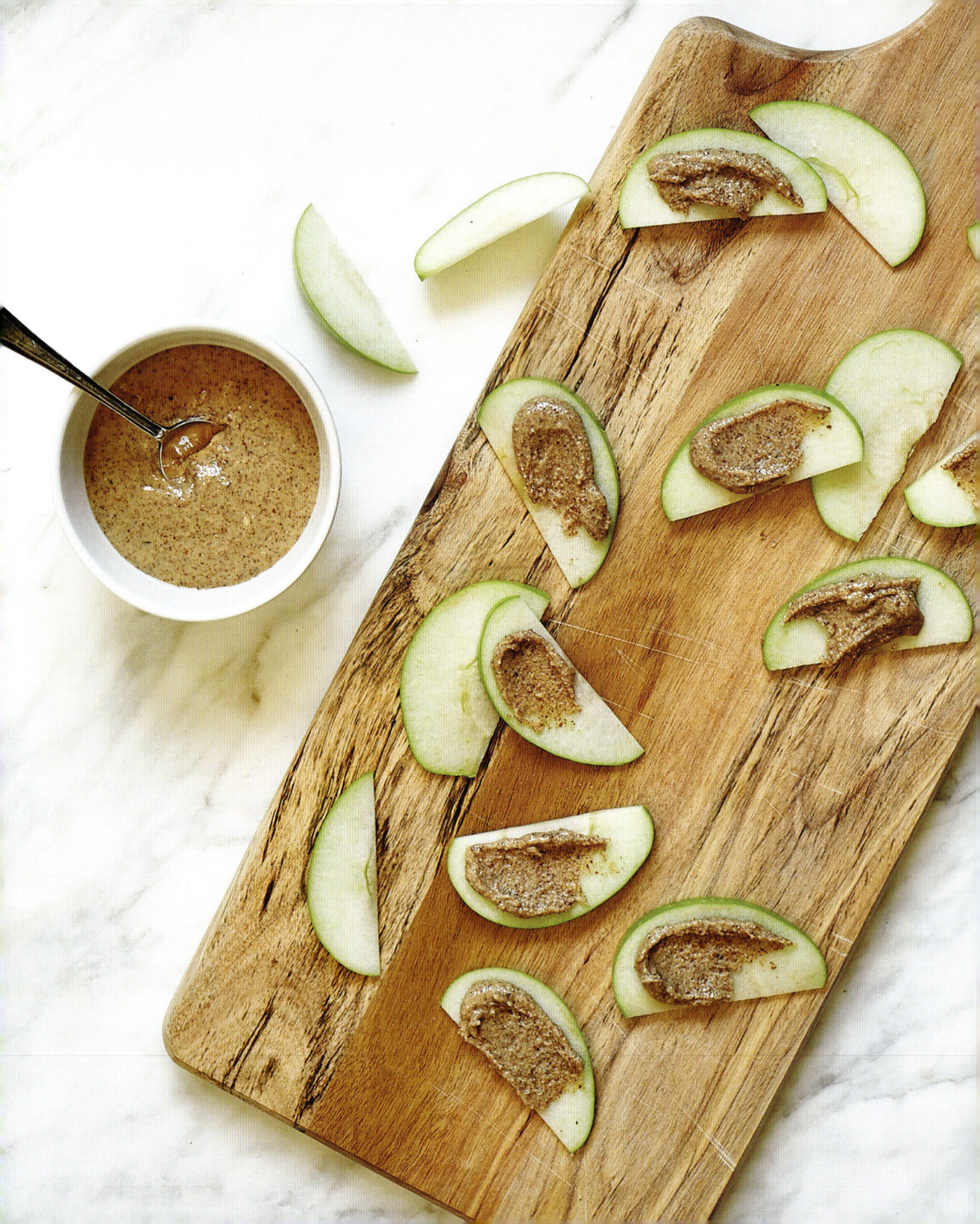

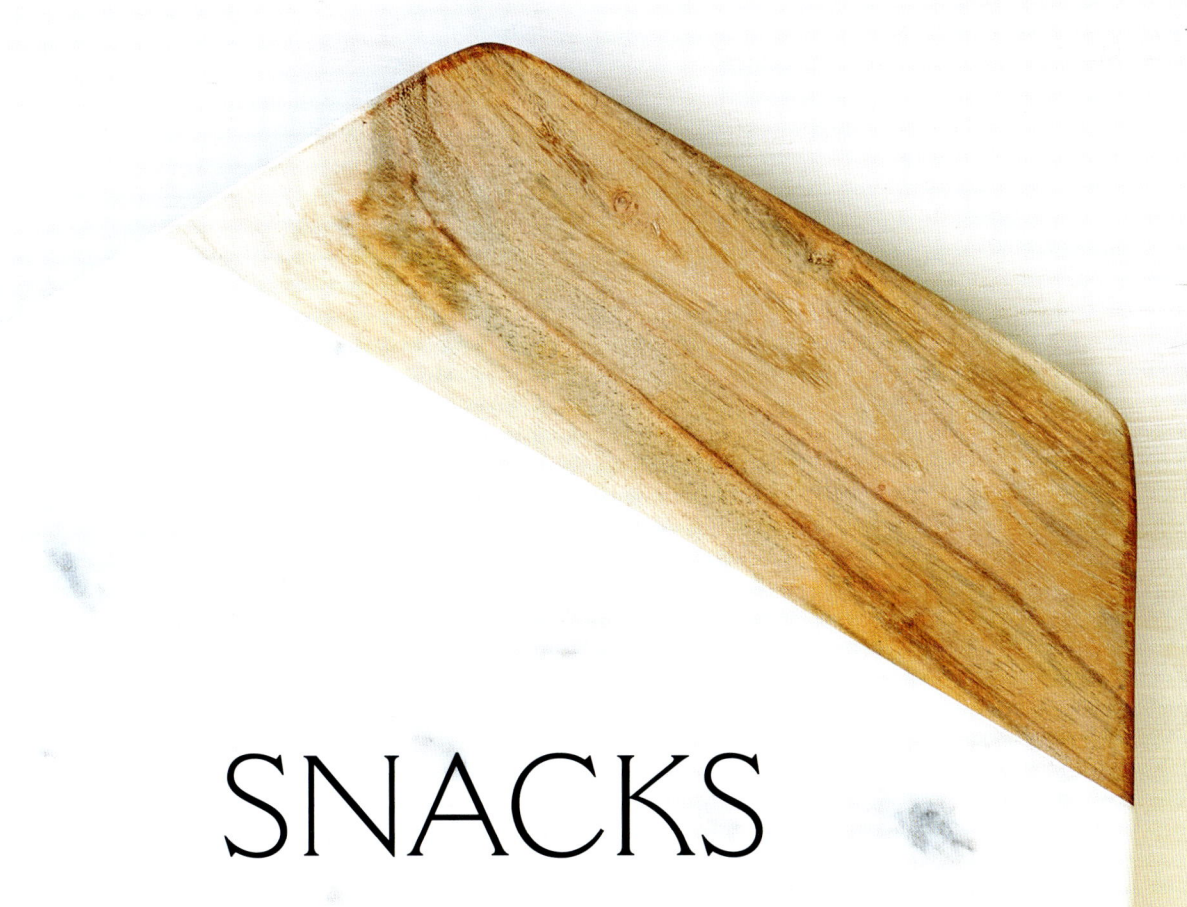

SNACKS

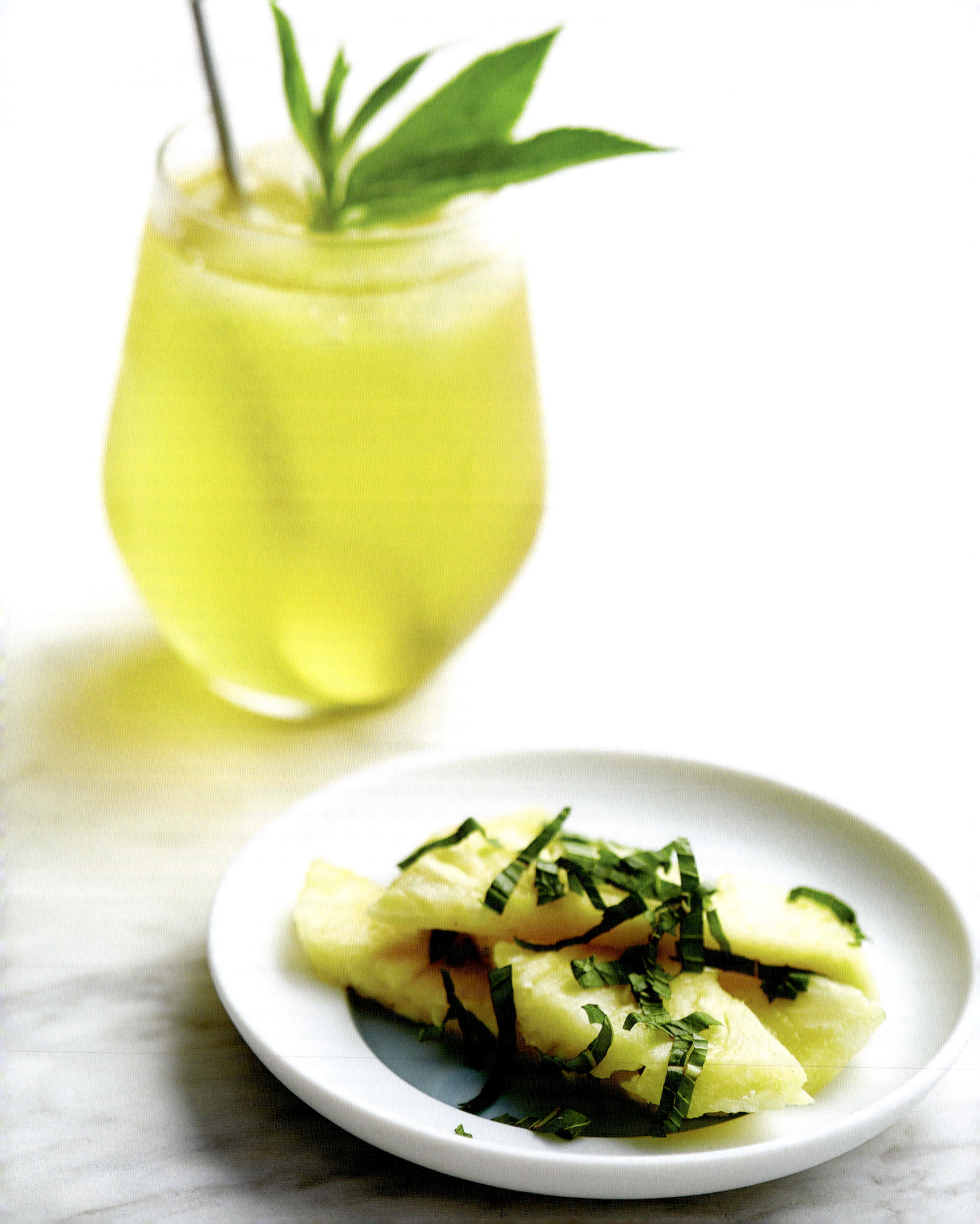

SNACKS

If you find you get hungry between meals and a glass or two of water is not stilling the hunger pangs, we have a great selection of healthy snack options that you can consider for your morning or afternoon break.

Medjool dates with brazil nuts
Take two or three fresh Medjool/Californian dates, remove the stone from each one, and replace with a Brazil nut.

Fresh pineapple with shredded mint
Take a fresh whole pineapple and, using a large kitchen knife, cut off the skin by running the knife down the side of the pineapple. Once the skin is removed, cut the pineapple into pieces, removing the hard core. Lay out on a platter. Finely chop some fresh mint and scatter over the top. It's so refreshing. Let everyone dig in or store in an airtight container in the fridge for 3–4 days, helping yourself to a few pieces, as needed.

Fresh apple slices spread with nut butter
Wash an apple and cut into thin slices. Spread some nut butter over part of each slice, and share with others. (Nut Butter recipe page 28)

Avocado with lemon juice
- » ½ ripe avocado
- » ½ lemon, juiced
- » salt and pepper

Cut the avocado in half lengthways, removing the stone and fill the cavity with lemon juice. Sprinkle with freshly ground black pepper and salt. Eat with a spoon.

Apple and brazil nuts
Wash and cut up a small fresh apple. Eat with 4 brazil nuts.

Edamame
- » 100 g (3 oz) frozen Edamame/soya beans in their pod
- » A big pinch salt

No need to defrost these edamame beans, they can be cooked from frozen. Follow the packet instructions for cooking or plunge into boiling water for 2 minutes, then drain. Run under cold water and drain again. Then put into a serving bowl and sprinkle over the salt. To eat, squeeze the beans out of the pods with your mouth and discard the pods.

A Big Mug Of Miso Soup
Keep some organic miso paste in your fridge and make up as per the packet instructions. This is a warming and sustaining snack, anytime of the year.

•Linseed and Pepita Rice Balls• Makes 10 balls

Packed with flavor, which stimulates your digestion, these balls are also a source of iodine to 'feed' your thyroid. Pumpkin seeds provide good levels of magnesium that help with blood sugar balance, relaxation and hormone balance. The fiber in the brown rice helps you to feel satisfied.

INGREDIENTS

- 10 g (½ oz) organic arame seaweed
- 3 tablespoons black and white sesame seeds, mixed
- 3 tablespoons flaxseed (linseed), freshly ground
- 3 tablespoons pepitas
- 400 g (14 oz) cooked short grain brown rice. About 200 g (7 oz) uncooked
- 2 pickled umeboshi plums, stones removed, finely diced
- 1 large spring onion (scallion), washed and finely sliced
- 2 heaped tablespoons pickled ginger, finely chopped (recipe page 35)

1. Cook the rice, if you don't have any already cooked. Note: It's important to use short grain rice as this, and the ground flaxseeds, make these balls sticky.
2. Soak the arame in water for 10 minutes. Once soaked, drain and finely chop.
3. Toast the sesame seeds and pepitas in a large dry frying pan/skillet, on medium heat, for a couple of minutes. Move the seeds around so they don't catch and burn.
4. Put them into a bowl. Add the seaweed, rice, plums, onion, ground flaxseed and ginger. Mix together well.
5. Wash your hands, leaving them a little moist. Take a tablespoon of mixture and roll and squeeze it into a ball in your hands. Repeat until you have used all the mixture.
6. These can be eaten straight away or wrapped and put in the fridge to be eaten the next day.

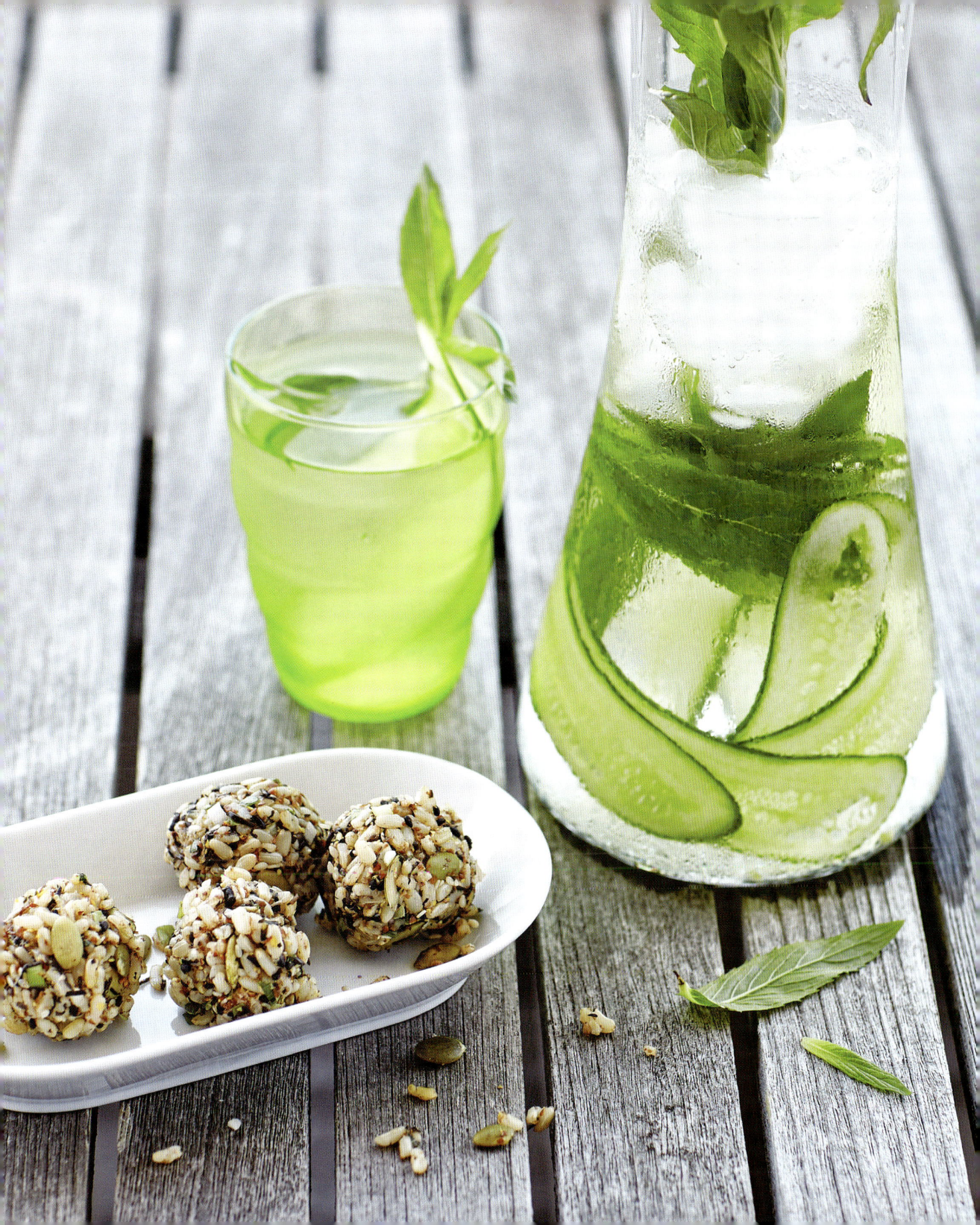

Lentil Falafels • Makes 15

These falafels are a good source of calcium, as well as fiber, which helps with bowel function and excretion of unwanted oestrogens. Lentils also contain iron, protein and folate. Folate helps produce the neurotransmitter 'good mood' hormones.

INGREDIENTS

- 65 g (2½ oz) raw pumpkin seeds
- 65 g (2½ oz) sunflower seeds
- 30 g (1 oz) sesame seeds
- 120 g (4½ oz) cooked orange lentils
- 20 g (1 oz) whole rolled oats
- 85 g (3 oz) tomato paste
- 1 heaped tablespoon tahini
- 1 heaped tablespoon fresh parsley, chopped
- Big pinch of cayenne pepper
- ½ teaspoon turmeric powder
- ½ teaspoon salt
- ¼ teaspoon freshly ground black pepper
- Extra sesame seeds, for covering

1. Set your oven at 160°C (325°F) fan forced or 180°C (350°F) regular, if baking the falafel.
2. Roast the pumpkin, sunflower and sesame seeds in the oven for 10 minutes. Or lightly toast the seeds in a large dry frying pan/skillet on medium heat for about 5 minutes, stirring them around frequently to stop them from catching on the pan.
3. Pour the seeds into a food processor mix for about 1 minute, to form a coarse seed grain. Then add the lentils, oats, tomato paste, tahini, parsley, cayenne pepper, turmeric, salt and black pepper. Blend until well mixed.
4. Form small balls (just a bit smaller than a golf ball) or patties with your hands. Roll with extra sesame seeds, if you want, and store in the fridge.
5. You can eat them just like this or bake them. If baking, place the balls/patties in the oven for 10 minutes. Turn or roll over and bake for another 5 minutes.
6. Eat hot or cold, dipped into Hummus (recipe page 184) or Tzatziki (recipe page 178).

Spicy Nut and Seed Crumble

Makes 8–10

In her clinic, Emma sometimes gets people saying they don't like eating plain nuts. So this recipe is for them! Nuts and seeds are high in good fats, minerals and protein. In particular, almonds contain beneficial levels of biotin and vitamin E, as do sunflower seeds, which are helpful in preventing both PMS and menopausal symptoms.

INGREDIENTS

- 150 g (5 oz) almonds
- 2 tablespoons black chia seeds
- 6 tablespoons sunflower seeds
- 1 teaspoon extra virgin olive oil
- 1 teaspoon salt
- 1 teaspoon smoked paprika (make sure it is smoked paprika)
- Big pinch of cayenne pepper
- 2 tablespoons tomato paste

1. Heat your oven 140°C (280°F) fan forced or 160°C (320°F) regular.
2. Mix all the ingredients together. Spoon them in clusters onto a baking tray lined with baking/parchment paper. Roast in the oven for approximately 30 minutes. Check every 10 minutes, shaking the clusters around to make sure they cook evenly.
3. Allow to cool completely, then eat straight away or store in an airtight container. This is a delicious crumbly mix of nuts and seeds.

•Tzatziki• Makes 400 g (14 oz)

Probiotic yogurt provides a good source of beneficial bacteria to help your gut to function well, absorb nutrients better and potentially improve both mood and female hormone balance. Use this tasty tzatziki as a dip or dollop onto salads or vegetables to add flavor.

INGREDIENTS
- 1 Lebanese cucumber, coarsely grated
- 1 large handful fresh mint leaves, washed and finely chopped
- 6 heaped tablespoons natural unsweetened organic yogurt
- 1 garlic clove, peeled and crushed
- ½ teaspoon ground cumin
- ½ lemon, juiced
- Pinch of salt

1. In a bowl gently combine the cucumber, yogurt, mint, cumin and garlic together. Don't over mix.
2. Pour into a serving bowl. Sprinkle the salt and a little extra cumin over the top. Drizzle with lemon juice and serve.

Carrot and Cumin Dip
Makes 700 g (25 oz)

This delicious dip contain lots of beta-carotene rich carrots, which once converted to vitamin A in your body, 'feed' your ovaries. The garlic is rich in prebiotic food and the yogurt contains good probiotic bacteria, both of which enhance your gut bacteria.

INGREDIENTS

- 3 tablespoons extra virgin olive oil
- 2 heaped teaspoons ground cumin
- 500 g (17½ oz) carrots, peeled and grated
- 2 medium garlic cloves, finely chopped or crushed
- A large pinch freshly ground black pepper and salt
- 200 g (7 oz) unsweetened natural goat or sheep yogurt

1. In a large frying pan/skillet, gently warm the cumin in the olive oil.
2. Then add the carrot and, on a medium/low heat fry, until soft, about 8–10 minutes. Stir in the garlic and pepper towards the end of cooking.
3. Allow to cool to room temperature. Once cooled, stir in the yogurt and sprinkle over the salt.
4. Serve with crunchy vegetables cut into bite size pieces. Raw fennel, celery, and snow peas (mange tout) are excellent with this dip. Or spread over homemade Sesame and Sunflower Crisp Breads (recipe page 181).

·Organic Chicken Liver Pate· Makes 350 g (12 oz)

Chicken livers are a really beneficial source of heme iron, the most easily absorbed type of iron for our bodies. Vitamin B12, which is very high in chicken livers, is a vitamin that is low in vegetarian diets. Vitamin B12 is important for female hormone balance. B12 is also used in energy production and liver detoxification.

Don't be put off by the idea of eating liver. This recipe is easy to make and is so good for you, especially if you are female.

INGREDIENTS
300 g (10½ oz) organic chicken livers, sinew removed
2 tablespoons extra virgin olive oil
¼ teaspoon freshly ground white or black pepper
A good pinch ground nutmeg
A good pinch ground cinnamon
A good pinch ground cloves
Pinch ground cardamom (if you have in your pantry)
1 small red onion, peeled and finely chopped
1 tablespoon finely chopped fresh thyme, plus a sprig for the top
1 garlic clove, peeled and crushed
¼ teaspoon salt

1. Cut away any white sinew on the chicken livers. It doesn't matter if you don't get it all. It can make the pate a little chewy.
2. In a large frying pan/skillet add 1 tablespoon of oil, plus the pepper, nutmeg, cinnamon, cloves and cardamom. Gently heat, then add the onion and cook on a low heat to soften.
3. Once the onions are soft, about 5 minutes, add the crushed garlic, stir around. Then put into a food processor.
4. Into the pan add the other 1 tablespoon of oil and the livers. Cook on a medium heat until the livers have almost cooked all the way through. To check this, pick the fattest one and, using a sharp knife, carefully cut it open. It should be a light pink on the inside.
5. Add the chopped thyme leaves and stir to combine. Then add the salt.
6. Once the livers are cooked put into the food processor with the onions and spices, and blend on high to form a smooth paste, about 30 seconds.
7. Add more oil if you need to, to get a smooth paste consistency that's not too thick or runny. You don't want it slipping off a spoon. Since you are making the pate with oil, it will not set much firmer than the consistency it is in the processor. Taste test to ensure the salt has blended through the mixture.
8. Scrape the mixture into a small ceramic pot/ramekin, smooth down the top. Add the sprig of thyme and pour a thin layer of oil over the top to prevent air from reaching the pate.
9. Cover the pot and place in the fridge to set, but importantly for the flavors to develop.
10. Eat spread over washed fresh celery stalks or Sesame and Sunflower Crisp Breads (recipe page 181)

   Notes:
   - If you don't like the pink color and are suspicious of it not being cooked enough, then cook the livers a bit more. The pate won't be quite as smooth as in a 5-star restaurant. The texture will be just fine and you'll be happier eating it.
   - You can also make this pate with organic butter instead of olive oil.

Sesame and Sunflower Crisp Breads
Makes 25

INGREDIENTS

- 5 tablespoons sunflower seeds
- 5 tablespoons black sesame seeds
- 5 tablespoons chia seeds
- 5 tablespoons flaxseed (linseed)
- 120 g (4½ oz) buckwheat or whole wheat flour
- 1 teaspoon sea salt flakes
- 60 ml (2 fl oz) extra virgin olive oil
- 125 ml (4 fl oz) water
- 1 tablespoon dried rosemary

1. Set your oven to 180°C (350°F) fan forced or 200°C (390°F) regular.
2. Mix all the ingredients together in a bowl using a spoon.
3. Tip the mixture onto a large baking tray (25 cm x 40 cm/12 inch x 15 inch) lined with baking/parchment paper.
4. Flatten out using the back of a spoon to as thin as possible, ideally filling the whole tray.
5. Bake in the oven for 25 minutes, then remove and allow to go completely cold before breaking up into portions.
6. These will store in an airtight container for a few weeks. If they go soft, put them in a moderately hot oven for 10 minutes to crisp up again.
7. Eat with Smashed Avocado (see page 73) or Hummus (see page 184) or crumbled into salads.

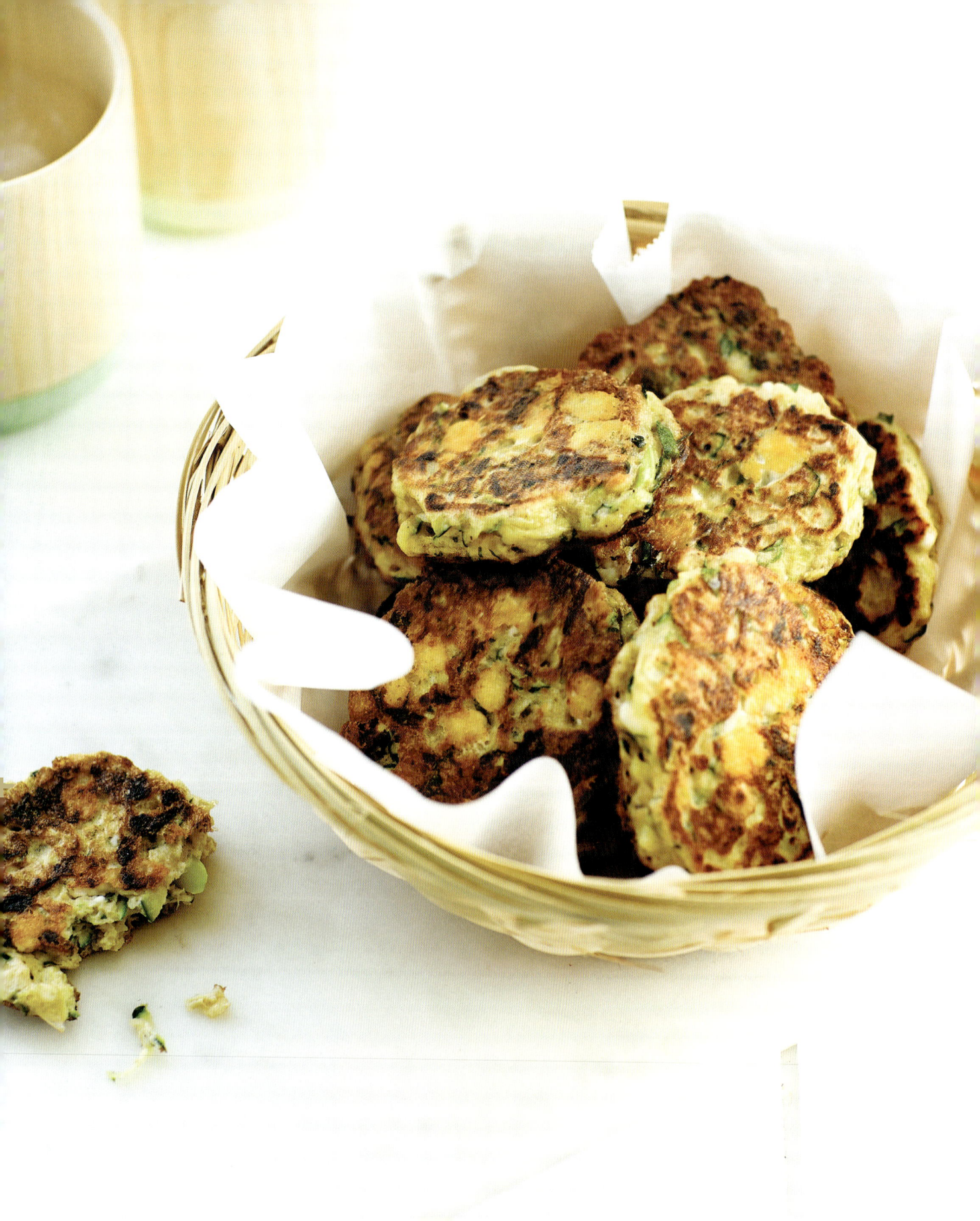

Green Zucchini Fritters
Makes 10 small fritters

Full of protein, good fats, phytonutrients and fiber, these little fritter snacks help to balance blood sugar and hormones.

INGREDIENTS
100 g (3½ oz) zucchini (courgette), coarsely grated
2 organic free range eggs
1 handful basil leaves, finely chopped
1 tablespoon flaxseed (linseed), freshly ground
80 g (3 oz) cooked chickpeas (garbanzo), roughly mashed
1 large spring onion (scallion), finely chopped
50 g (2 oz) goat or sheep feta, crumbled
Big pinch of salt and freshly ground pepper
1 teaspoon extra virgin olive oil or organic butter
1 lemon

1. Mix all the ingredients, except the oil/butter, together in a bowl.
2. Brush a large frying pan/skillet with some oil/melted butter and bring to low heat. Add dessert spoons of the mixture to the pan.
3. Cook until the mixture begins to brown and set, about 1 minute, then flip the fritters, and cook on the other side for 30 seconds. You want the egg to cook and go firm.
4. Squeeze over some lemon juice or dip into Tzatziki (recipe page 178).

Hummus with Cumin and Garlic *Makes 300 g (10 ½ oz)*

Chickpeas contain isoflavones, which are a source of phytoestrogens. These phytoestrogens help relieve symptoms such as PMS, acne, weight gain and menopausal conditions. They also contain fiber, which assists your body to clear unwanted oestrogen.

INGREDIENTS
230 g (8 oz) cooked chickpeas (cook your own or canned)
½ garlic clove, peeled
2 tablespoons tahini
1 small lemon, juiced
2 tablespoons extra virgin olive oil
1 teaspoon apple cider vinegar
2 heaped teaspoons ground cumin
½ teaspoon salt
20–30 ml (½–1 fl oz) liquid from the chickpea cooking or can

1. If cooking your own chickpeas, cook until just soft.
2. Put all the ingredients into a food processor and blend until creamy in texture. If too thick, slowly add more water until you have the desired texture.
3. Check the seasoning. Add more salt, cumin, lemon juice, if you like.
4. Ideas: Dress it up by adding fresh or dried herbs, such as basil or coriander, if you have some. Or add a small cooked beetroot.
5. Store in the fridge for a couple of days or freeze.
6. This humus is even better the following day, once the flavors have developed.

Flaxseed and Parmesan Oatcakes
Makes about 15–20

These nutritious oatcakes are a great source of soluble and insoluble fiber, helping to keep your gut and liver happy.

INGREDIENTS
100 g (3 ½ oz) whole rolled oats
120 g (4 oz) seeds - pumpkin, sesame and sunflower
20 g (1 oz) flaxseeds (linseeds)
Big pinch of cayenne pepper
50 g (2 oz) freshly grated Parmesan cheese
Big pinch sea salt flakes, plus ½ teaspoon for decorating the top
50 ml (1 ½ fl oz) extra virgin olive oil
5–6 tablespoons water

1. Preheat your oven to 180°c (350°F) fan forced, 200°c (375°F) regular.
2. Put all the seeds and oats into a food processor and blitz until they form a crumb, but not until they are as fine as flour.
3. Add a big pinch of salt, the oil, cayenne, cheese and water and blend until a ball of pastry-like dough is formed.
4. Tip this onto the bench top with a large piece of baking/parchment paper below it.
5. Put another piece of baking/parchment paper over the top and using a rolling pin or similar, roll out until the dough is about 5mm (¼ inch) thick, if wanting thin crisp oatcakes, or 1.5cm (½ inch) thick for softer thicker oatcakes.
6. Sprinkle ½ teaspoon of sea salt flakes over the top of the rolled dough.
7. Use a 4 cm (1 ½ inch) or 5 cm (2 inch) cookie cutter to cut out the oatcakes or, using a sharp knife, cut out similar sized squares.
8. Line a large baking sheet with baking/parchment paper and place the oatcakes onto it. Line them up quite close together since they will not expand. Once all the oatcakes are on your tray/s, put them into the oven to bake for 15 minutes if thin, or 20 minutes if thicker.
9. Allow to cool completely before moving.

NOTE: These are great eaten as a snack or they go well on the side with some home made soup.

ACKNOWLEDGEMENTS

We thank all the women in Emma's clinic who have challenged her to make a difference in their lives.

We especially thank our families, friends and all the people who have cooked, tried, tested, tasted and enjoyed all the recipes in this book. Their support, feedback and ideas have contributed in both small and large ways. We are grateful to them for the part they have played in bringing this book to you.

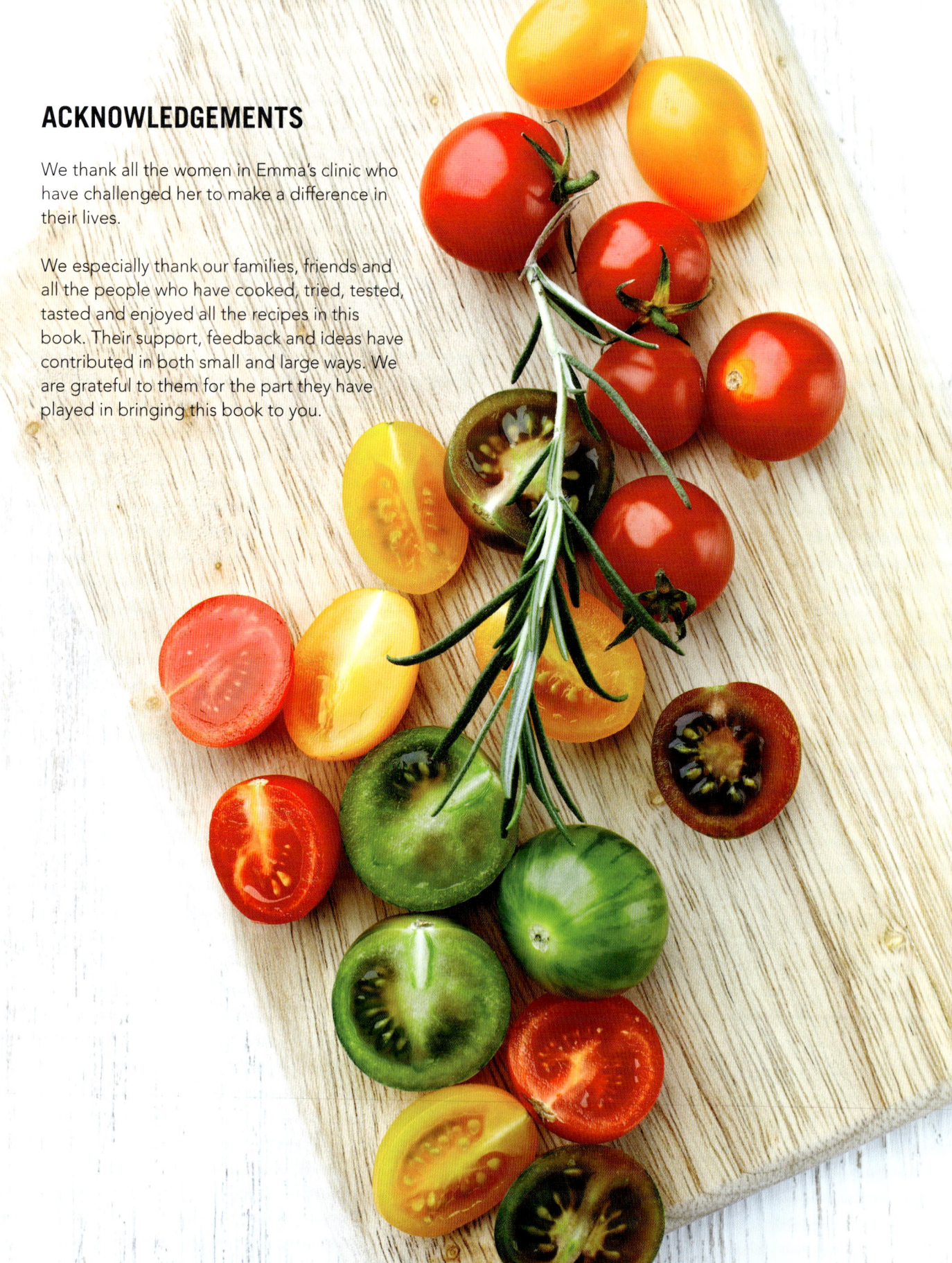

INDEX

A
Alcohol 10
Anti-Inflammatory Foods 10
Apple
    Apple and Cinnamon Flapjacks 52
    Apple and Fennel Slaw 80
    Apple with Brazil Nuts 173
    Fresh Apple Slices with Nut Butter 173
Avocado
    Home Cured Salmon with Avocado 59
    Falafels with Avocado and Oregano Salad 69
    Smashed Avocado with Chickpeas, Feta and Lime 73
    Avocado and Lemon Juice 173

B
Balance 11
Banana, Power-packed Banana Bites 146
Beef
    Bone Broth 27
    Oh-So-Slow-Cooked Beef with Sweet Potato 120
    Seared Beef with Lime, Lemongrass and Coconut Salad 129
Black Bean and Mushroom Stew 115
Black Rice Porridge 38
Bone Health 12
Breakouts and Maintaining the Habit 13
Burgers, Chicken and Lentil 81
Buying Fresh and Buying Local 13

C
Cakes
    Divine Chocolate Cake 155
    Strawberry and Coconut 147
Calamari, Spicy Calamari with Okra, Avocado and Black Beans 106
Cauliflower
    Chana Masala 134
    Pickled Turmeric Cauliflower 34
Chicken
    Bone Broth 26
    Chicken and Lentil Burgers 81
    Fragrant Larb Salad 137
    Mint and Bean Salad with Polenta Chicken 133
    Organic Chicken Liver Pate 180
Chocolate
    Divine Chocolate Cake 155
    Hot Chocolate 168
    Mousse 152
    Orange and Cacao Balls 143
    Truffles 153
Coffee
    Coffee and Caffeine 158
    Iced Coffee 159

D
Dates, Medjool Dates with Brazil Nuts 173
Digestion 14
Dips
    Carrot and Cumin 179
    Hummus with Cumin and Garlic 184
    Tzatziki 178
Drinks
    Fermented 161
    Not So Favourable 161

E
Edamame 173
Eggs
    Green Egg Pies 63
    Lentil Cakes with Poached Eggs 49
    Puttanesca Green Beans and Broccoli with Poached Eggs 83
    Ranch Eggs with Spinach 55
    Spanish Style Tortilla with Mushrooms 60
Exercise and Movement 14

F
Falafels
    With Avocado and Oregano Salad 69
    Lentil Falafels 176
Fats, Good 16
Fermented Drinks 161
Flapjacks, Apple and Cinnamon 52
Fiber 15

Fig and Ginger Slice 149
Fish
   Cakes with Sweet Potato Chips and Red Cabbage Slaw 113
   Home Cured Salmon 32
   Salmon with Avocado 59
   Sesame Crusted Salmon with Asian Slaw 109
   Roast Cauliflower with Mediterranean Salsa and Snapper 110
   Wombok, Asparagus and Mushroom Salad with Salmon 114
Flaxseed Meal 30
Flesh 15
Fruit Salad, Warm with Nut Crumble 144

G

Gardening 16
Ginger
   Pickled Ginger 35
   Zesty Lime and Ginger Balls 140
Grains 17
Gut Health 18

H

Hormone Disruptors 18
Hormone Imbalance 9
Hummus with Cumin and Garlic 184

I

Ice cream, Mango and Flaxseed Soft Serve 150

J

Juice, Cleansing 162

L

Labne 33
Lamb, Parsley and Quinoa Tabouli with Lamb 124
Liver Health 19

M

Mindfulness 20
Muesli
   Berry Bircher Muesli 41
   Jill's Digestive 48

Mushrooms
   Black Bean and Mushroom Stew 115
   Field Mushrooms with Saffron Yoghurt 56
   Harrisa-crusted Mushrooms with Lentil, Pomegranate and Eggplant 116
   Mushroom and Buckwheat Noodle Salad 78
   Quinoa Crusted Mushroom Pie with Wilted Greens 119

N

Nuts
   Nut Butter 28
   Nut Milk 29
   Spicy Nut and Seed Crumble 177

O

Oats
   Chai Tea Porridge 42
   Coconut, Oat and Black Rice Porridge 44
   Amaranth, Oat and Mushroom Porridge 45
   Pink Oats 47
   Overnight Berry Oats 53
   Flaxseed and Parmesan Oatcakes 185

P

Pancakes, Buckwheat Pancakes with Smashed Berries 51
Parsley Oil 75
Pate, Organic Chicken Liver 180
Phytoestrogens and Soy Foods 22
Pineapple with Shredded Mint 173
Porridge Three ways 42
Prawns, Wok-tossed Prawns, Spinach and Brown Rice 102

R

Rice
   Black Rice Porridge 38
   DIY Rice Paper Rolls with Avocado and Mint 88
   Ginger and Edamame Turmeric Fried Rice 93
   Linseed and Pepita Rice Balls 174

S

Salad
   Apple and Fennel Slaw 80

Fragrant Larb Salad 137
In A Jar 66
Mushroom and Buckwheat Noodle Salad 78
Parsley and Quinoa Tabouli with Lamb 124
Preserved Lemon and Olive Salad with Labne 77
Ruby Grapefruit and Mint 91
Roast Pumpkin and Olive Salad with Haloumi 130
Roasted Beetroot and Cauliflower 135
Ruby Grapefruit and Mint 91
Wakame Seaweed with Crunchy Tofu 94
Warm Beetroot, Chickpea and Red cabbage 97
Watercress and Mango Salad with Turmeric Prawns 105
Watercress, Broccolini and Walnut 87

Sesame and Sunflower Crisp Breads 181
Sleep 22
Smoothies
    Summer Berry 164
    Thick Chocolate and Chia 165
    Super Green 167
Soups
    All-Things-Green Warming Broth 70
    Big Mug of Goodness 92
    Big Mug of Miso Soup 173
    Carrot, Leek and Borlotti Bean Soup with Parsley Oil 75
    Nourishing Broth with Ginger and Wild Mushrooms 74
    Salmon and Turmeric Broth 98
Sprouted Pulses 31
Stress 23
Sugar 23

T

Tart, Red Onion Tart with Herb Salad 84
Teas 160
    Ginger and Mint Iced Tea 160
    Medicinal Herbal 160
Turmeric, Iced Turmeric Milk 169
Tzatziki 178

V

Vegetables, Baked Vegetables with Smokey Paprika 123

W

Water 158
Where to Shop 25

Z

Zucchini, Green Zucchini Fritters 183

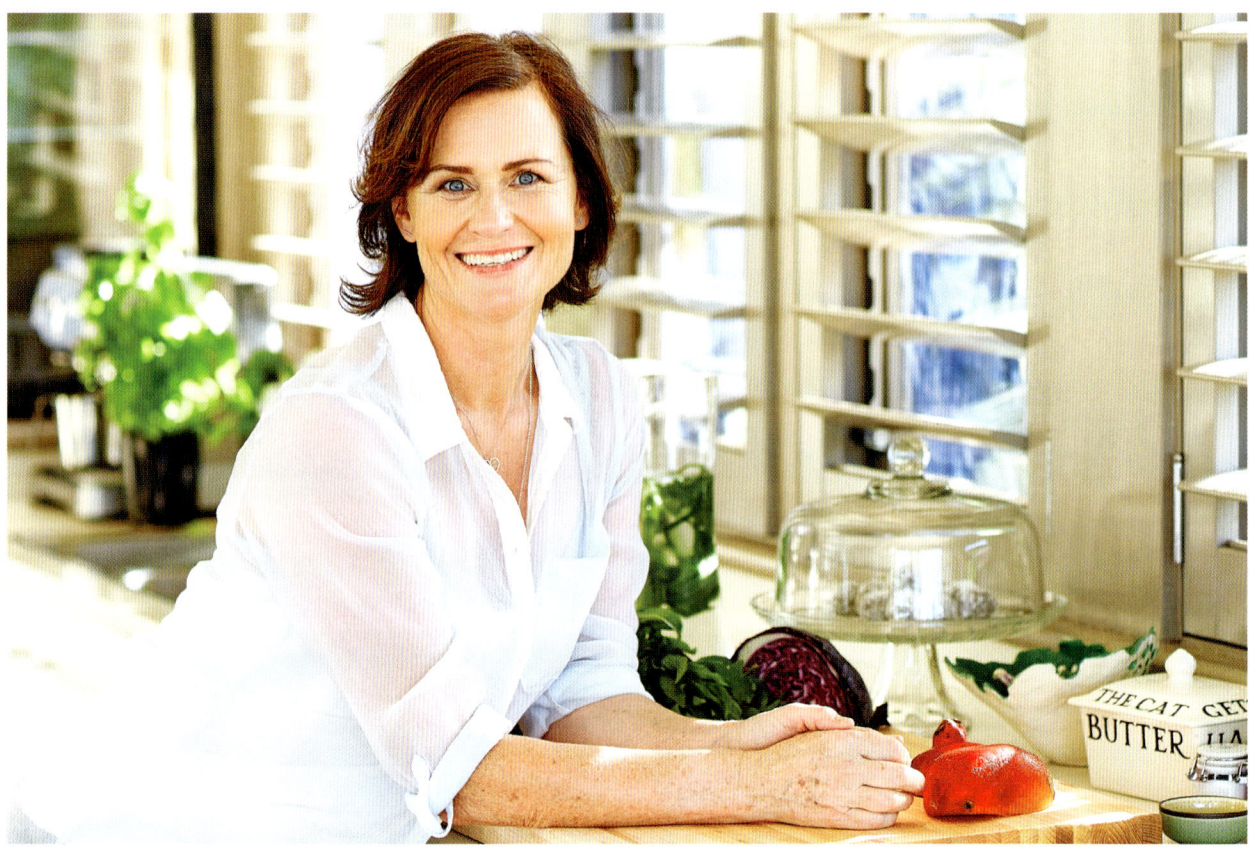

PROFILES

Emma Ellice-Flint

Emma brings to this book, not only a number of years of clinical experience and evidence-based nutrition, but a wealth of knowledge about food and an excitement that goes with that understanding.

Her own personal research led her to see a gap in accessible information about how to manage and balance female hormones. This book helps to fill that gap for women of all ages.

"I am so excited to have written this female hormone balance cookbook. I am often asked for recipes in my clinic work. This is where the passion for improved health and change comes about, from a person's eating. It makes the difference."

Before qualifying and working as a nutritionist, Emma worked as a chef both in London and Sydney. She currently practices at Eatcetera Nutrition in Sydney, Australia.

Emma has a Bachelor of Health Science degree in Nutrition. She regularly attends ongoing professional education.

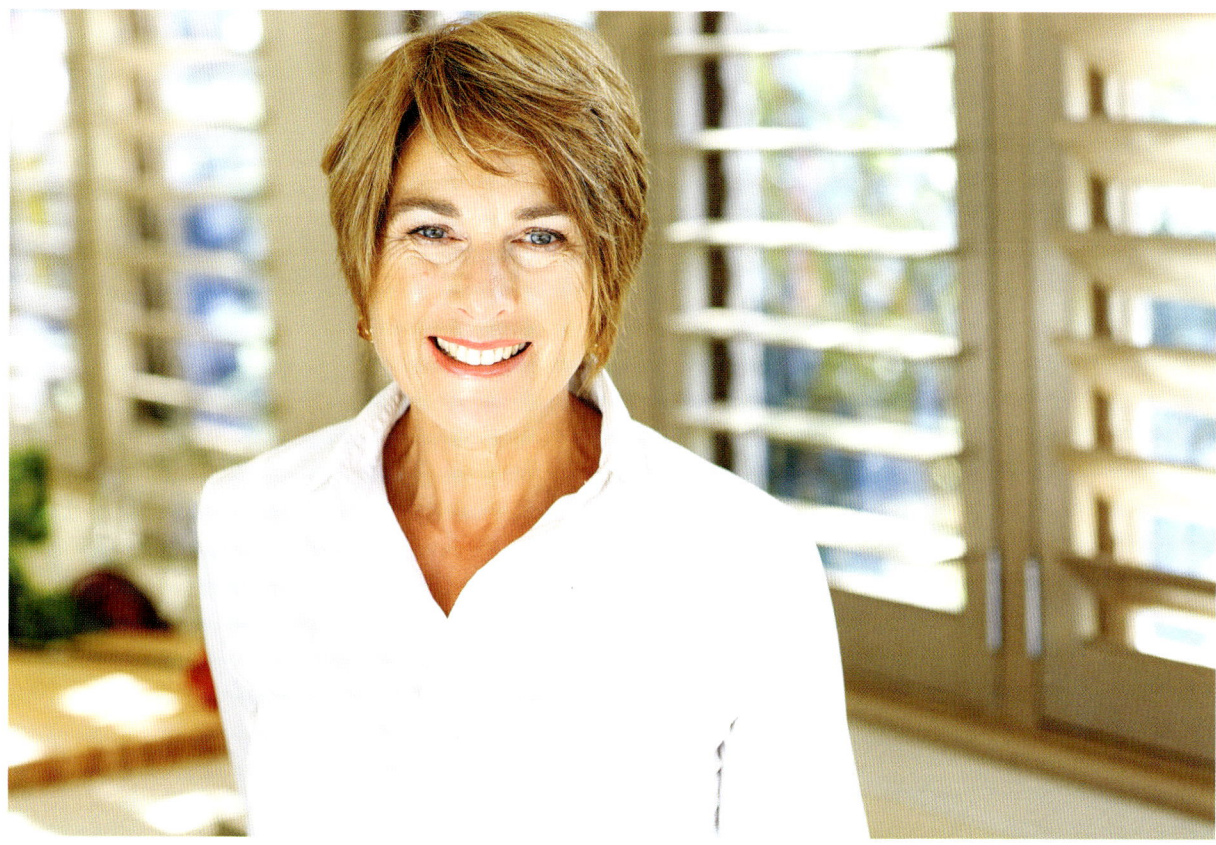

Jill Keyte

Jill has been interested in health and what makes us healthy all her adult life.

Some years ago she had a real need to look at what was happening with her hormones. She consulted Emma Ellice-Flint and made some changes to an already healthy diet. These changes had a very positive impact on her wellbeing – more energy, better sleep and uplifted mood.

After a brush with early breast cancer, she decided to follow an eating plan that would keep her hormones happy naturally. Jill has been enjoying Emma's recipes for some years now.

Jill's professional background is in arts and event management. In 2015 and 2016 she ran a series of healthy cooking workshops and weekend retreats involving Emma under the banner, The Vital You, which takes a holistic approach to living - caring for the physical, emotional, mental and spiritual. Jill is studying nutrition.

She is a keen gardener, cook, bushwalker and yoga practitioner. Good healthy food, exercise and mindfulness are central to her life.

First published in 2016 by New Holland Publishers

London • Sydney • Auckland
The Chandlery, 50 Westminster Bridge Road, London SE1 7QY, United Kingdom
1/66 Gibbes Street, Chatswood, NSW 2067, Australia
5/39 Woodside Avenue, Northcote, Auckland 0627, New Zealand

www.newhollandpublishers.com

Copyright © 2016 New Holland Publishers
Text copyright © 2016 Emma Ellice-Flint & Jill Keyte
Photography © 2016 New Holland Publishers
Shutterstock: pages 3, 8, 86, 122, 186, 187 and 192

All rights reserved. No part of this publication may be reproduced, stored in a retrieval system or transmitted, in any form or by any means, electronic, mechanical, photocopying, recording or otherwise, without the prior written permission of the publishers and copyright holders.

A record of this book is held at the British Library and the National Library of Australia.

ISBN 9781742578682

Managing Director: Fiona Shultz
Publisher: Diane Ward
Editor: Gordana Trifunovic
Designer: Lorena Susak
Photographer: Julie Crespel
Stylist: Imogene Roache
Production Director: James Mills-Hicks
Printer: Hang Tai Printing Company Limited

10 9 8 7 6 5 4 3 2

Keep up with New Holland Publishers on Facebook
www.facebook.com/NewHollandPublishers